<u>About the author</u>

Ross A. Wright is a father, good friend, respected attorney, part-time
professor, martial artist, and community activist. He has worked in
corporate legal departments of the General Electric Company and Convergys
Corporation managing complex commercial transactions, negotiation,
litigation, and compliance among other areas. He began his legal career as
an Assistant Prosecuting Attorney in the Hamilton County Prosecutor. s
Office, and prior to that he worked at Taft, Stettinius & Hollister L.L.P.
where he worked as a litigator.

Ross is an Adjunct Professor both at Xavier University (MBA program) and
also the University of Cincinnati (business law). Mr. Wright holds
B.B.A., M.B.A., and J.D. degrees (1986-1994) from the University of
Cincinnati. He currently serves on the River City Correctional Facility
Governing Board, and Hamilton County Public Library Board. Ross.
hobbies include: Quality time w/family and close friends, Brazilian Jiu
Jitsu (black belt), biking, building solar + wind energy contraptions,
traveling, reading, nutrition, fitness and overall living life to the
fullest.

1

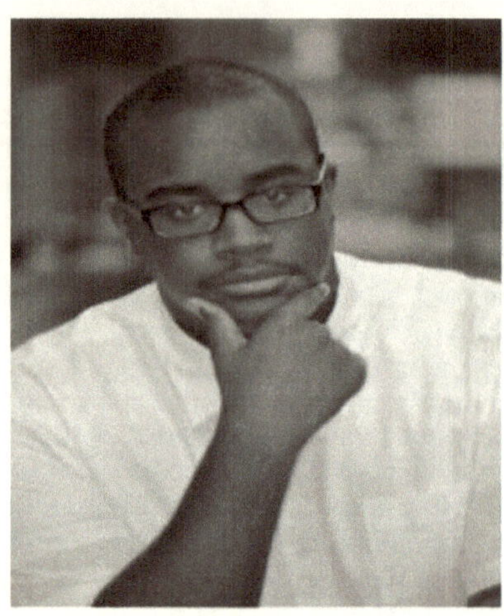

Bilal Wright: Bilal is WOMP's Vice-President of school pursuing a career in Robotics & Engineering. Bilal graduated from Sycamore High-School in 2014. In addition to his duties at WOMP, Bilal works full time as a engineering tech, trustee of the Patricia D Wright Foundation, landlord/property owner, investor, and volunteers periodically at the Freestore Foodbank and Little Brothers Friends of the Elderly. Bilal enjoys traveling, outdoors, reading, sports, and video games in his spare time.

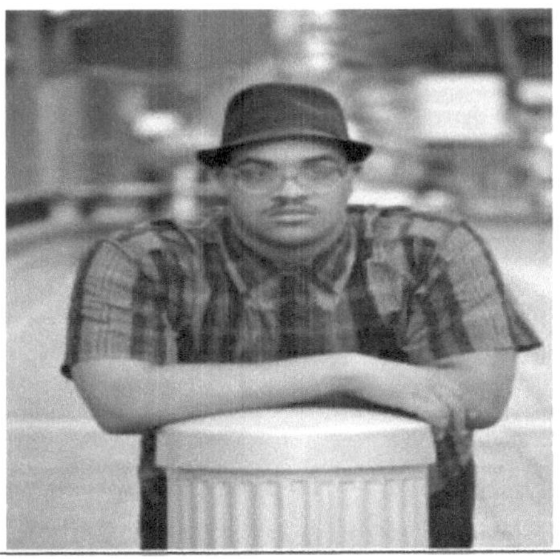

Malachi Wright: Malachi is WOMP. s Vice-
Malachi is pursuing a career in customer service. Malachi graduated from
Sycamore High-School in 2014. In addition to his duties for WOMP,
Malachi works full time as a customer engagement specialist at a large
retail company, trustee Patricia D Wright Foundation, landlord/property
owner, investor, and volunteers periodically at the Little Brothers
Friends of the Elderly and Freestore Foodbank. Malachi enjoys traveling,
outdoors, movies, reading and computers in his spare time.

<u>*THE TABLE OF LIFE PLANNING:*</u>

1. <u>Father-Dad:</u>   A key ingredient of a productive society

2. <u>Spirituality:</u>   Your bushido for doing good

3. <u>Simple Living:</u>   The art of hanging loose in a uptight world

4. <u>Wellness=Nutrition + Fitness:</u>   Living with zest

5. <u>Life success:</u>   Find what you love, love what you do

6. <u>A Life Plan:</u>   "Do or do not there is no try!"

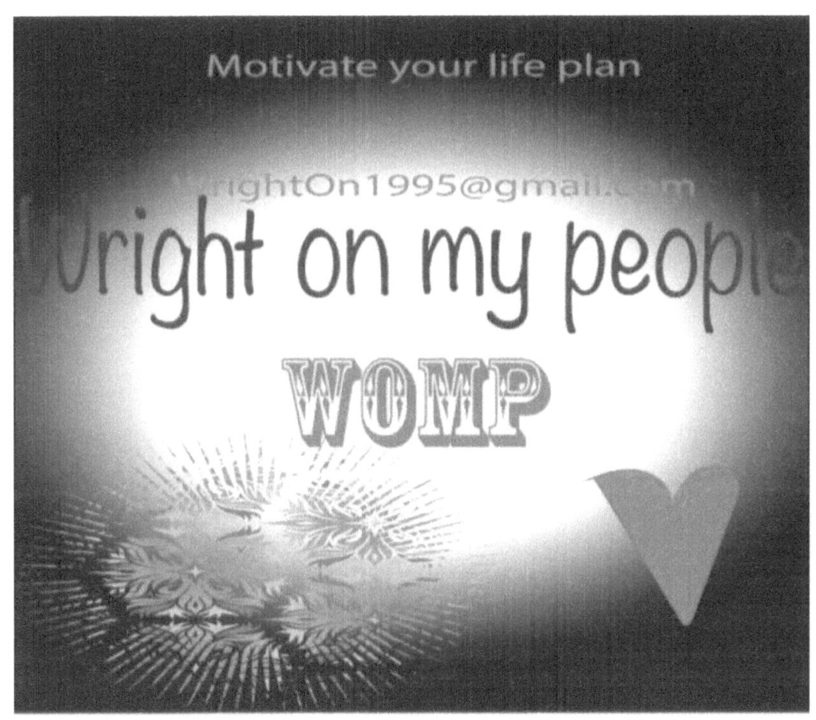

Artwork designed by Malachi A. Wright

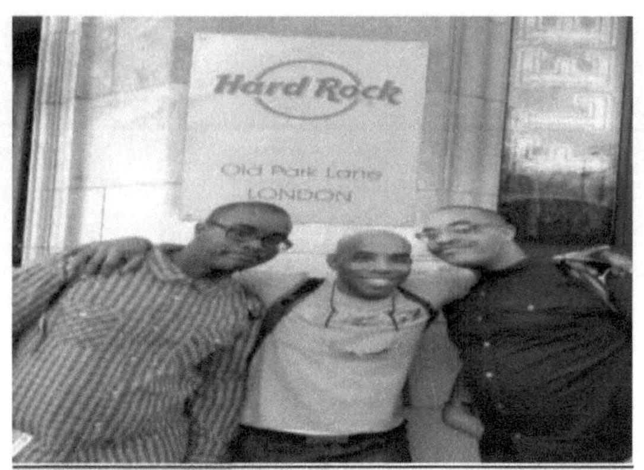

London, England 2014:
High-school graduation celebration and international learning
experience

FOREWORD:

Social media is used by millions of people daily all over the world to drive a variety of behaviors, some good and some bad. Under the auspices of Wright on My People LLC, my sons and I are publishing this compilation of living tips in our first e-book. Our purpose is to highlight those elements of our life that we believe lead to robust and productive citizenship by chronicling our journey through social media since 2007. We believe this sharing of valuable life tools can be used to facilitate positive change across a broad spectrum of human behaviors including fatherhood,

spirituality, 6

fitness and nutrition, simple living, personal finance,
professional success and accomplishing your goals by
developing a life plan.

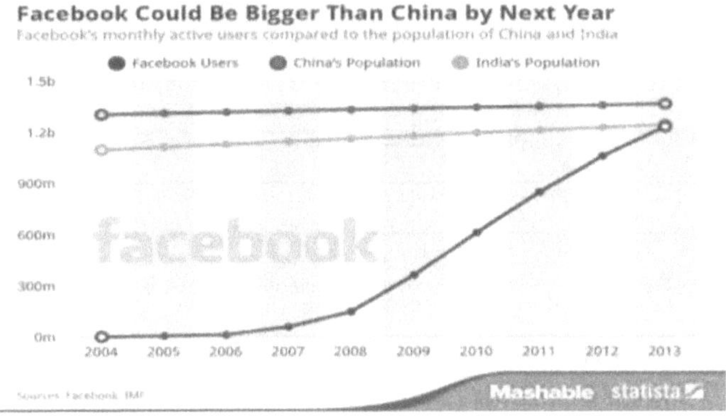

The chart above demonstrates the impact of social media on the world
In this life, we can easily be lulled into the idea that
someone else will be the " change agent" and dispense the
gifts the Universe has bestowed upon us. It. s always
somebody else who is better, never us. The Scriptures tell us
" prophet is not without honor except in their own land,
among their own people. " This simply means we may be one of
those people who can provide the change or do great things,
but sometimes the people in the closest proximity to us do not
recognize or encourage our potential while others will

see that potential.   It's always ʼ that person ʼ over in
there in the secret temple, or the person coming on the magic
carpet with magic dust that going is to fix everything.
WOMP's message is the answer to our problems is within us if
we do enough introspection to find it.   Now, this sounds
cliché and many people will read this and say, ʼ Yeah, yeah,
and yeah!ʼ   My answer to this kind of subtle negativism is:
ʼ excessive pessimism is the mother of the non-achiever ʼ .

WOMP rejects preconceived notions and false
constructs of what supposedly has to be.   What has to be
is what ʼ we make it ʼ . Just because we're young
doesn't automatically mean we have to engage in
excessive amounts of dumb behaviors.   We can teach our
young to be wiser much sooner.   Just because someone is
nearly 50 years old doesn't mean that person has to be
broken down, on numerous prescription medications, obese
and unhealthy.   Just because someone is poor or black or
disadvantaged in any way doesn't automatically you will
fail in life.   We all have gifts to show forth to the
world if we only quiet our minds to find our gifts.   We
are then called upon to use those gifts to raise our own
consciousness and that of the people around us to advance
humanity.

Since May 19, 1995, the date my sons came on this planet, I. ve told both my sons that they have the power and potential to change the reality of this world, starting with their immediate surroundings. Many people do not know this, but both my sons have their own set of personal challenges. Malachi is high functioning on the Autistic Spectrum and Bilal is on the high functioning side of Asperger. s Syndrome.

Now, we could have just thrown in the towel and conceded that these challenges would knock them out of the ball game of life-low educational achievement, job prospects, independence as an adult, low achiever and overall just not very productive as a citizen. Despite what some of the medical tests showed when they were two years old, there was never any worry that Malachi and Bilal would not or could not succeed in life. Both have faced their challenges, worked extremely hard and have far exceeded expectations of what many thought was possible. And now, there are two blossoming, educated young men who will make a positive contribution to this society. This e-book is a manifestation of that and as they say, ˅ The proof is in the pudding!˯

My son Malachi around 7 years old once told me he was
considering making a spaceship and wondered if I would fly
with him to Neptune.   I answered Malachi by saying, " If I
have enough vacation time, then I. ll definitely go with
you. ,   Now detractors will say, " You. re endorsing
unrealistic expectations and creating a
formula for failure, .   I disagree.   I was creating a mindset
that would allow my son. s brain to expand beyond his current
state of being.   As Malachi and I discussed in future
conversations the engineering and physics involved in a trip
to Neptune, Malachi realized the spaceship idea may not be
viable.   So Malachi came to the realization that he may not
want to do exactly that, but his creativity to do new things
was preserved and nurtured.   That is what good parenting is!
As my sons grew, I would periodically remind them of why they
bore the names they have, more positive reinforcement.   This
was another reminder of their potential and worth to me as
human beings.

> _My words to Malachi_: " Malachi, you. re named after the
> last prophet in the Old Testament whose is referred to
> as " My Messenger, and the " M, as your first initial
> means YOU have the power to be magnificent and do
> magnificent things in this life, .

My words to Bilal: Bilal, you have a North African name. The person you are named after was tortured to renounce his belief in the One God, which the historical Bilal refused to do. The "B" as your first initial means YOU have the capacity to be brilliant like the Sun, so always remember to shine your light to the world.

The origins of this mentality are embedded in the great family legacy from which we emerge. Our ancestors Samuel Ross Wright (grandfather), Amanda Beatrice Scott (great grandmother), George Hannibal Wright (great grandfather), Patricia D. Wright (mother), and Victoria Holloway-Wright (Aunt), and many other aunts, uncles and cousins serve as the platform upon which Wright On My People was conceived and built. The torch of their wisdom has been genetically and spiritually transmitted to us. As inheritors of this great legacy, we decided to share our life experiences via this e-book.

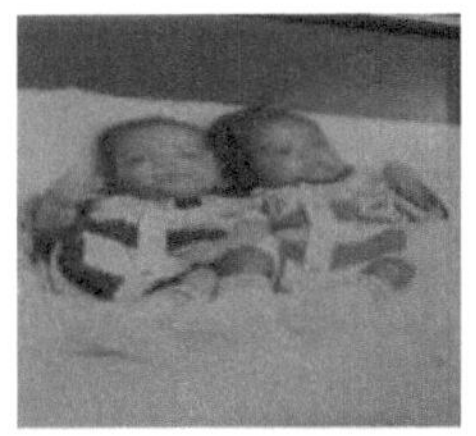 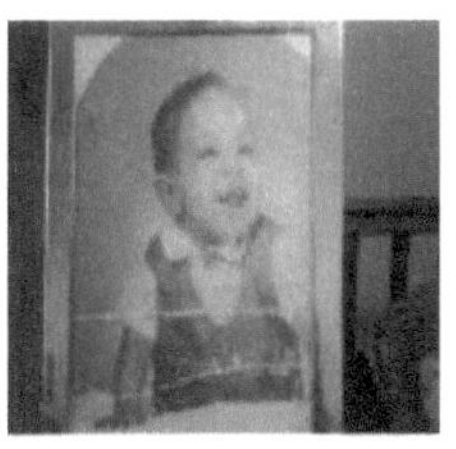

Malachi & Bilal Wright   Ross A. Wright

This e-book represents a compilation, organization and
dissemination of our message as shared on Facebook and other
social media platforms over the past eight years. We expect
you to extract tangible benefits from this e-book that will
have an objectively
measurable positive impact on how you live your life going
forward.

Our philosophy is positive change starts right where we are.
We seek to inspire by our living example, goals,
visualization, and impactful positive messaging.   While we
do not endorse any specific religious dogmas, we do adhere to
universal principles that permeate many of the established
religions across the world. In the final analysis, what
truly matters is not how often we went to church, synagogue
or temple, but how we allow our personal moral code and/or
spiritual beliefs to positively impact our fellow travelers
in the human experience. Many of the chapters to follow are
built upon " DAD Talks® , which represent a series of
conversations between my sons and me addressing core issues
we face in society over their 20 years of life. Other
chapters are simply reflective of what we call the Wright On
My People living experience.

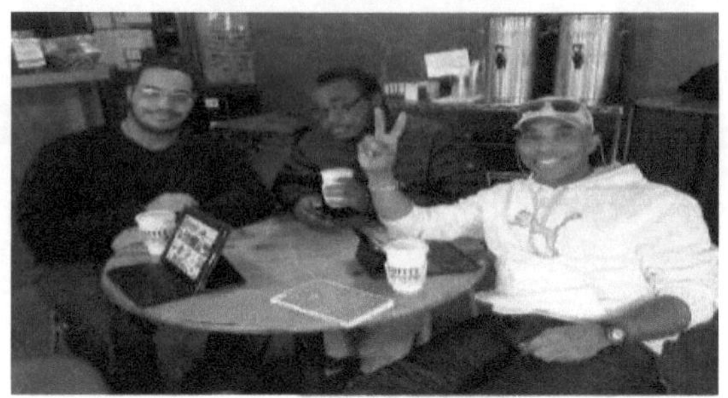

Weekly café connection

CHAPTER 1: "FATHER-DAD"

o *Fathers, do not provoke your children to anger, but bring*

> *them up in the discipline and instruction of the Lord.*

> *(Ephesians 6:4)*

o *A father should be careful to keep his son from lies, and*

> *he should always keep his word to his children.*
> *(Talmud*

> *Sukkah 46b)*

o *A father is equivalent to a hundred professors.* –
Hindu

> *Scriptures (Manusmiriti)*

o   *When you teach your son, you teach your son's son.* –

> *Talmud*

o *"Your God has decreed that thou shalt worship only Him*

> *and adopt good behavior with (thy) parents.*
> *(Qur'an,*

17:23)

The term " father " can take on various meanings, both symbolic and literal. The definition we prefer to use for this book is its literal use: " A male, whose sperm unites with an egg, producing an embryo and that male' s relationship to his natural child. "   A step above " father" is " dad" . A " dad" is a father who *is integrally involved in the continued development of their offspring into a productive citizen, providing love, discipline sprinkled with compassion, wisdom and guidance.* Our term " Father-Dad" combines both concepts. The " Father-Dad" concept requires robust communication, compassion, discipline and being the example in how we conduct our own affairs, because our children are watching!

I was reared by a single mother (Patricia D. Wright) with the help of my extended family, most notably my grandfather Rev. Samuel Ross Wright, and aunt Victoria Wright Holloway. My mom was a 20-year-old student at the University of Cincinnati, majoring in psychology when she became pregnant with me. She was a very intelligent woman, but got involved in a relationship which ended up in a less than ideal situation for her-unmarried, not finished with college, and pregnant with child. Under these circumstances and understandably so, many advised my mother against keeping me.

And early in her pregnancy, I was slated to be adopted by a
family in the greater Little Rock, Arkansas area. Pursuant
to that path, my mother finished the last few months of her
pregnancy in Little Rock to side step the judgmental
commentary of folks regarding her being a pregnant, unmarried
daughter of a minister.

As the Universe and the course of history would have
it, my grandfather Rev Samuel Ross Wright wrote my mother a
beautiful, inspirational letter encouraging her to be a
great mother. That letter (some simple, yet profound
words on a piece of paper) helped turn the tide of history
in favor of my mother keeping me. And 47 years later,
history bears witness that my mother made the correct
decision. Absent my mother's decision to keep and rear me,
the people I've been able to touch, including that of my
sons, may have never happened. I thank the Almighty God
every day for my
mother's choice to keep me, as well as, the collective
support from my extended family to develop me over the
years. And to this day, I've never had a relationship with
my physical father, but I had the fathering of my
grandfather, uncles and cousins to mold me into the man I
became. I've taken that collective fathering influence and

channeled it into my own brand of fatherhood to give to my
sons.

16

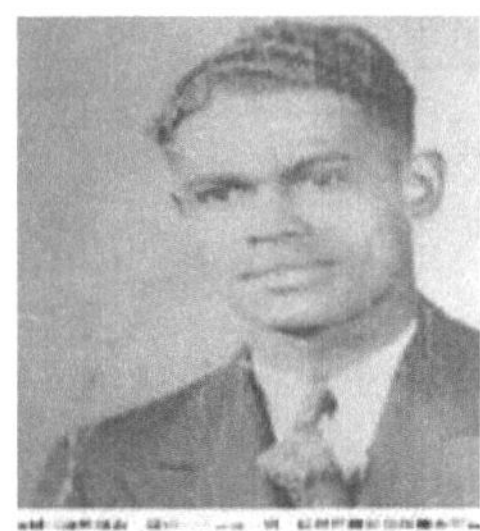

Samuel Ross Wright,

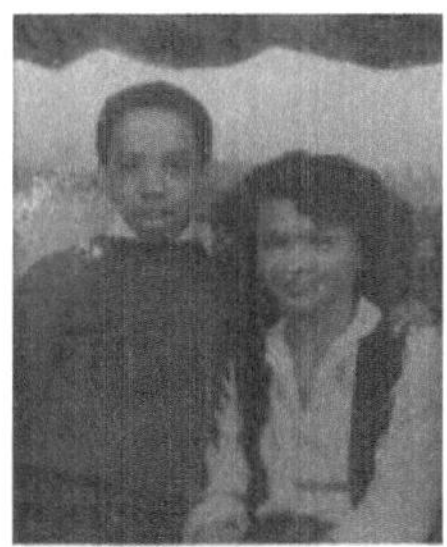

My mom and I

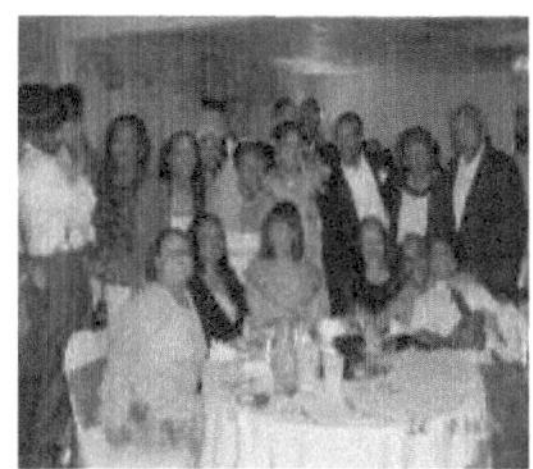

Family photo

The ⸰ Father-Dad⸰ concept does not mean we are perfect,
but we invest quality time in our children, other than just
sporting, entertainment and other perceived ⸰ fun events⸰ .
The Father-Dad is a nurturer who enables his children to go
farther...FA-⸰ R⸰ -THER !
We. ve got to bring the same enthusiasm to social
responsibility, ethics, and spiritual development as we do
to our favorite sports teams.   In addition, the sole
allocation of household responsibilities 17

by gender is unintelligent. As fathers and sons, we can
learn to cook, clean and manage household duties. My mother
was a big proponent of this concept. If you dirty up
clothes, you can wash them. If you eat, you can cook. This
makes us more balanced and appreciative of the work required
to manage a house. And we can still watch sports, go camping
and engage in other activities
earmarked as " manly, in our society. In terms of driving
these behaviors and other positive behaviors on social media,
I. ve summarized various verbal conversations and advice to
my sons in social media writings, which are called, " Dad
Talks, .

My sons listen to me through these Dad Talks, not
because I. m a lawyer, not because I drive or want a certain
kind of car, live in an over-sized house, nor is it due to my
job title at work,
checking/saving account balance, but it is because I
sincerely give them my time, my brain, my love and
chastisement, when needed, to advance their growth. And the
number one reason they listen, above all else, is they watch
me to see how my actions match my words, doing otherwise is
the textbook definition of hypocrisy.

18

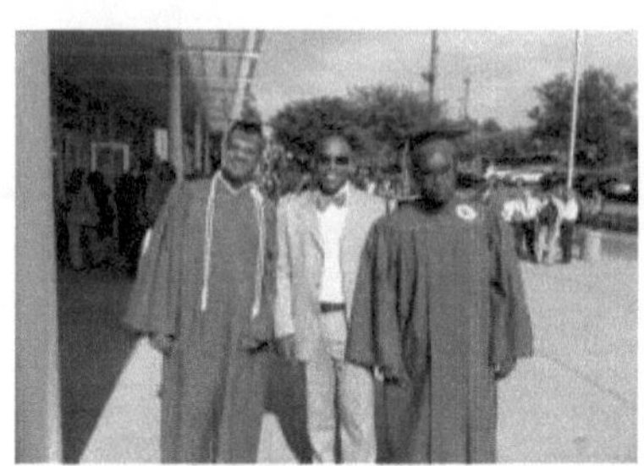

[*] Education is the key to success. - Rev. Samuel Ross
Wright, (WOMP patriarch)

<u>DAD TALKS</u> [Prepare for your future]: Once I shared with my
sons the story of "the ant v. the grasshopper": "So fellas,
one of my favorite Bible books is Proverbs, because Proverbs
addresses the practicalities of living versus deep, esoteric
spiritual concepts, which are also needed. Even though there
is science that suggests the average life expectancy of a
grasshopper may exceed that of the ant, the more important
takeaway of the comparison is to work hard, work smart v.
being lazy, and don. t live entirely in the moment with no
prep for the future or a future generation of species. Each
generation of

grasshoppers generally dies, although eggs are laid for the
next generation. No history is passed down to tell the next
generation of grasshoppers, "prepare for winter!. The ants,
unlike the

grasshoppers, do a much better job of that. Ants are always

19

methodically working away for the next generation of ants

knowing that the winter is coming. I'm an ant and you are the

next generation of ants. As you grow in knowledge and wisdom,

enjoy and live in the moment to a reasonable degree, but have

the mentality of the ant by preparing for your future."

(Proverbs 6:6-8; 30: 27)

DAD TALKS [Education Audits]: So those who know anything

about my parenting style know that I am good for a "roll up"

on my sons without notice, sometimes at school or elsewhere.

I. m like a surprise auditor who shows up to see how things

are going. I

performed some notorious "roll ups" on my sons during their

entire elementary, junior high-school and high-school

educational lives, and it hasn't ended post high-school. As

your grandfather once told me, " Education is the key!" A

key is that which opens doors. Education has allowed me to

choose my profession /career versus having a career imposed

upon me due to the lack of education or training. If you

desire to have control over your career and not work a 20

year old job at 50 years old, then education should be a

complete area of focus for you. Sure, while you are on your

path, you will work less desirable jobs, but those jobs are

just stepping stones to your ultimate career. Education will

empower you to manage your life in so many

ways, so don. t skimp on it, nor relegate yourself to the short term benefit of a job that is far below your potential.

Expressed in " Father-Dad" math: parenting presence, love and wisdom > material gifts.

The Universe works like a bamboo tree in that it is firm, yet pliable enough to adapt and make adjustments. You must be the same way to succeed!

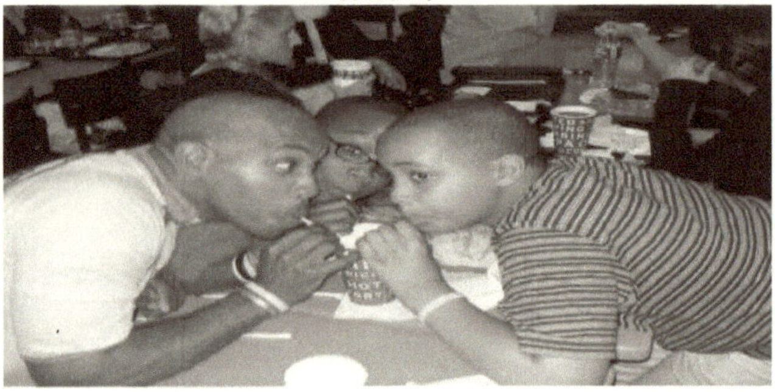

Wright on My People, spreading the knowledge and fun in Times Square, New York City, Café Europa

DAD Talks (Be the Renaissance Person): Fellas, another success factor in life is being MULTI-dimensional versus a ONE dimensional human being. We live in a specialized society, which has its benefits with expertise in certain subject matters. However, strive to be that person whose expertise spans a significant number of different subject areas. You can do it. In other words, always have some key

areas of focus/expertise in life, but be in a perpetual state of learning and growth over a range of topics. For instance, it is great to have passion around a topic like sports. I love football, basketball, Brazilian Jiu Jitsu, tennis, etc..., but if the diameter of your thinking is solely limited to just sports or any one topic, then the circumference of your activity will keep your brain in a small, uninspired circle.

This requires you to have an unquenchable thirst for knowledge. And not just the knowledge to pay your bills or advance your career, but learning for the sake of learning with no financial rewards or achievement medals attached to it. So if you can't have a meaningful conversation about a broad range of subjects that encompass this thing we call living, then you have no depth=ONE dimensional.

Read, study, experience, interact and learn from everyone in your circle about many different topics to apply to your life. Never be that person who is like a walking trivia show that knows lots of things, but doesn't apply their knowledge to their own life to improve it. And don't be that person with one million ideas, none of which this person spends one ounce of energy trying to bring into reality.

[3] The diameter of your thinking controls the circumference of your
activity. Be a modern day Imhotep and Da Vinci in your sphere of
influence, a
renaissance man ![8]

22

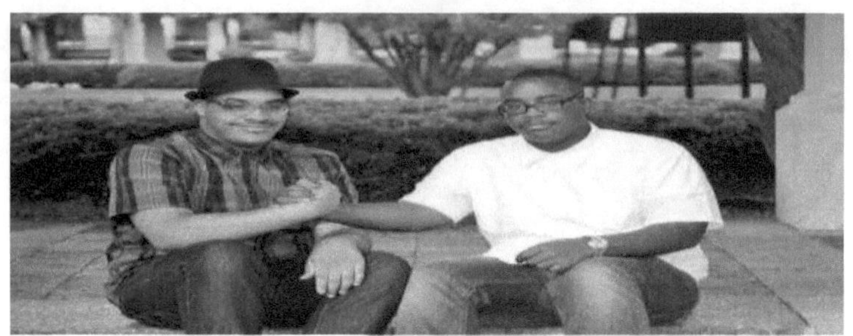

Renaissance men in progress, Wright On!

Dad Talks [Make decisions]: So fellas of the many Bible verses quoted by people, one of the most frequently misinterpreted and partially quoted verses are the following, "Judge not, that ye be not judged. 2 For with what judgment ye judge, ye shall be judged: and with what measure ye mete, it shall be measured to you again." Matt 7:1-2.   Many people use this quote to cop opt of making a decision citing " We. re not supposed to judge. . Wrong! The second verse which provides, "For with what judgment ye judge, YE SHALL BE JUDGED, AND WITH WHAT MEASURE YE METE, IT SHALL BE MEASURED AGAINST YOU" is ALWAYS left out of the citation even though the person using the quote is hoping to stifle your

23

decisiveness while holding themselves out to the world as a
Bible expert. The combination of both verses above permits
judging with the understanding that the standard of
"judgment" you use towards something will also be applied to
your own conduct. The verse does NOT say, "Don't judge". Why
doesn't it say that? Because
underneath EVERY decision we make in life each day is a
"judgment" (clothes we wear, church/religion we embrace, our
political
philosophy, what profession we chose, what sports we like,
who we decide to hang around socially, our nutrition and
exercise, etc...].
When we make a choice on any life decision, we are JUDGING
the alternative options to choose one option we judge to
be the best option.

So in your dealings with society fellas as you make
various life decisions in politics, on social issues, job
choices and others, although you may be shunned or isolated
by a segment of the community for speaking your truth, always
be as collaborative as possible, but make a dammed decision.
And to those who continually evade the
decision under the mirage " don. t judge. rule, here is a
proposed response: "With all due respect, we make judgments

every moment of each day of our life, so please don't attempt

to admonish me by

24

partially quoting a Bible verse that it seems you haven't even fully read. If you are too timid to take a firm position on an issue or speak your truth, then I regret to inform you I don't suffer from that same communication malady." In making reasonable judgments, use compassion mixed with common sense.

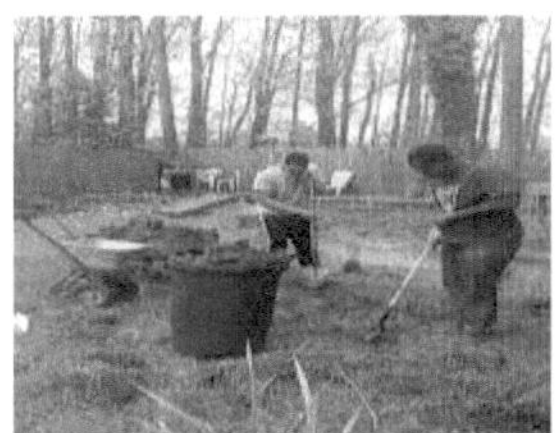
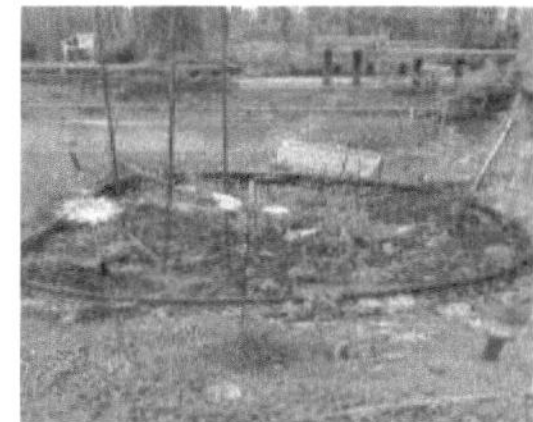
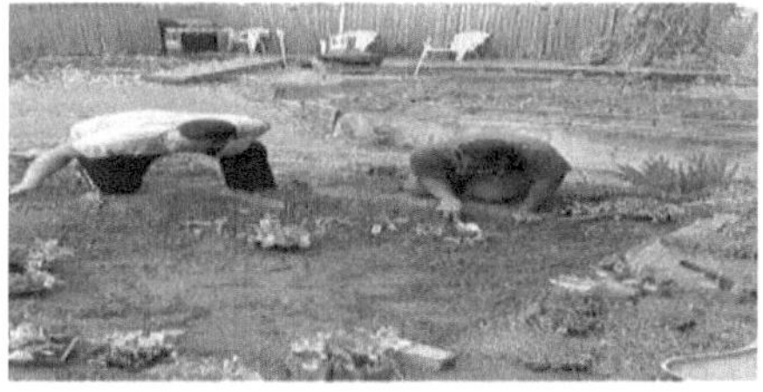

Wright On My People. s veggie garden: in life, we reap what we sow

<u>Dad Talks</u> [Assessing People]: So in my daily five minute conversations with my sons, one of them asked me "Dad, how do you evaluate people?" Me: [paused and had to give that some thought]:

25

"Well, here are a few of my "people metrics", which you can apply to see how they work for you:

1) How much do they generally desire to learn through books, electronic and/or print media, etc... regarding things of substance v. Hollywood fantasy, excessive TV, or other mindless activities?

2) How resolute are they to their professed core living principles? For instance, are they resolute to their professed core principles in your presence when surrounded by an audience of people who want then to do something opposite of what they claimed to you they believed in private? If the person caves, or their knees buckle under the societal pressure to their professed principles, know that in times of controversy, adversity or storm, this person is NOT to be heavily relied upon.

3) Does the person keep their word the majority of time or is their word as flimsy as a house of cards? If you use these three metrics and assign an evaluation score to the subject person(s), you will save yourself much

agony, disappointment and distress and build
strong friendships by weeding out the
unreliable. And oh, by the way, you need to be
performing at 90+ percent on the same three
metrics before you can use them for evaluation
of others.

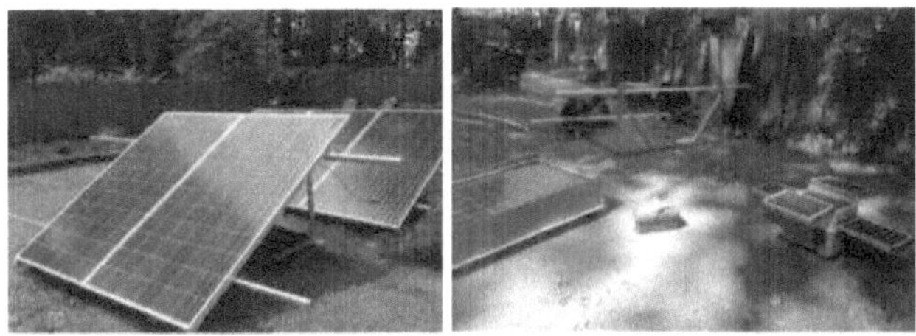

Malachi and Bilal help install solar panels at our home, go green !

DAD Talk [GIVE YOUR BEST]:   My sons asked me yesterday,
"Dad, you're spending a ton of time preparing for this
Brazilian Jiu Jitsu World Championship, what if you don. t
win?   Me: "Good question. Jiu Jitsu is like life, there are
no guarantees. I've certainly won more than I've lost in
competition, but more important to me is preparing to win,
something I have control over.   If I make a mistake or my
opponent is simply better, I can accept and respect that, but
I have no tolerance for not preparing to win.   In your life
endeavors, you should do the same...prepare to win physically
and mentally".

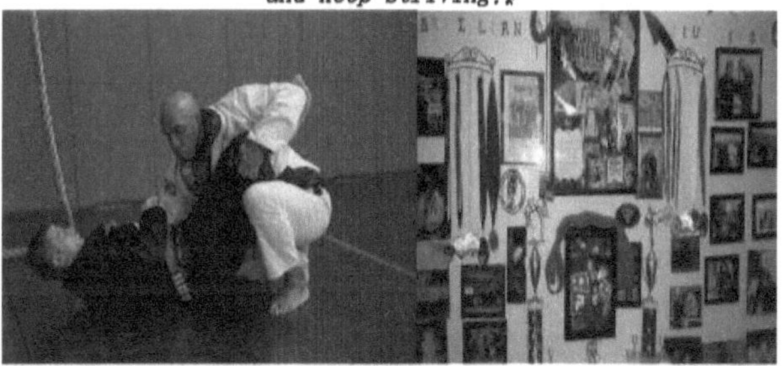

Training Brazilian Jiu Jitsu, a life passion for me

<u>DAD Talk {Where did the time go?] Time accountability:</u>   So this is
an exercise I use with my sons whenever they don't get a task
complete or complete the task in a non-timely fashion allegedly for a
"lack of time" to do it.   Fellas, there are 168 hours in a week. Of those
168 hours, a reasonable person allocates time as follows:

Sleep: 8 hrs. per day=56 week (some only get 6-7)
Work: 8 hrs. per day=56 week (some less or more)
Exercise 1 hrs. per day=7 week (some less)
Meals and bathroom 2 hours per day=14 per week (some less)
TV 2 hrs. per day=14 per week (some less=me)
Miscellaneous stuff: 1 hour per day= 7 per week (some
less)

Total=154 hours accounted for out of 168 hours in a week

Where. d the time go?   So we can safely say that the average person
likely has 10 to 15 hours per week of unaccounted for time, so go find

28

those hours brothers and get your task list completed on
time. You can either reallocate the existing hours from the
above list of activities or engage in better time
management/calendaring/organizational rigor of the
unaccounted for time. But with my frenetic schedule that
I. ve had for 20 years or more, "your lack of time" excuse
falls on deaf ears. And the only person who is going to take
responsibility for the time in your life is you. And how you
chose to allocate your time is critical in the process. Our
society wastes hours of time watching EXCESSIVE amounts of
stupid TV shows, playing and doing other mindless activity.
We all need a release, but in reasonable doses. If you are
allowing key components of your personal development lapse
due to being consumed with dumb, time wasting activities,
then you will get dumber, be less productive and be in less
of a position to help facilitate change in society. I. m a
big proponent of individual freedom, so the choice is yours
ultimately. Time is a precious gift. It is not guaranteed,
so use it wisely and make the most of it to achieve your
goals, which we will discuss in Chapter 6, " Life Plan" .

Summary

There is no pre-set path to being a successful Father-Dad.
Having never had the involvement of my biological father, I
never had a true "Father-Dad" in the form of my biological
father. As I mentioned, my "dads" were my grandfather,
uncles, older cousins and elders in the community who showed
me the example of Dad in how they reared their children.
The most important ingredient to the Father-Dad relationship
is consistent engagement in every aspect of your child. s
life combined with meaningful communication and face to face
connection versus texting only. Our children determine who
we are by what we do, not what we say. Sounds simple right?
It astonishes me how parents live a life completely
contradictory to the life they advise their children to
live, yet expect something different from their children.
Children and young adults are a lot smarter than we give
them credit. They see the hypocrisy, so we parents are not
pulling a fast one on them as we may naively think.
If we want our children to read, we should read. If we want
to be financially responsible, we have to be. If we want our
children to

meditate, pray and live a spiritual life, we have to do the same. My great grandfather George Hannibal Wright was reputed to have said, " How can I hear the words coming out of your mouth when your actions keep thundering in my ears?" Let our lives as parents reflect the values we want in our children, because this encapsulates the Father-Dad concept.

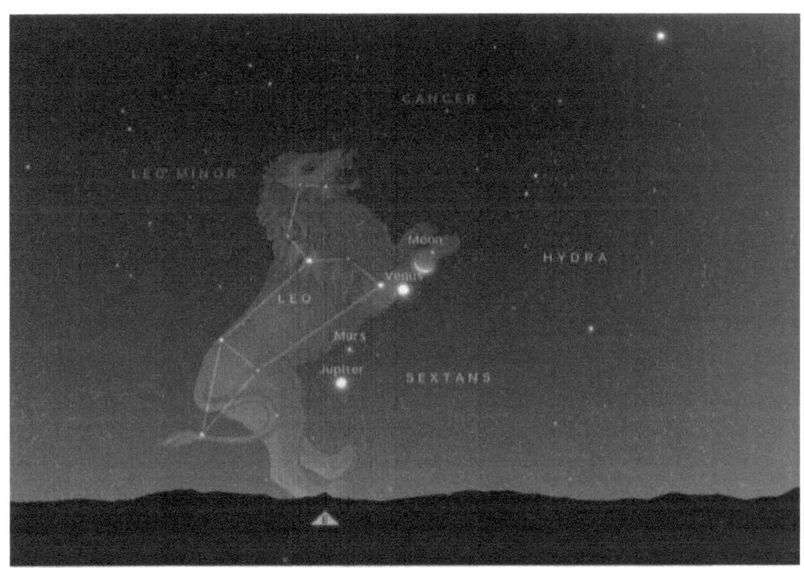

Astronomy: A Wright On My People recommended activity

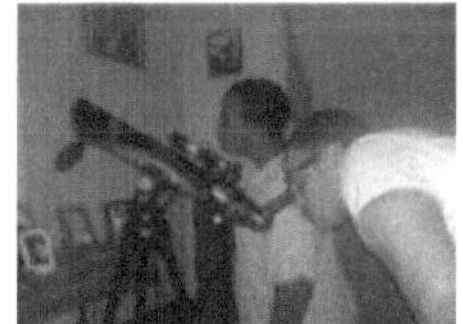

A fair number of us grew up with some form of
religious or some ⁼ ism⌐ : Christianity, Islam, and
Judaism, Hinduism, or Buddhism.

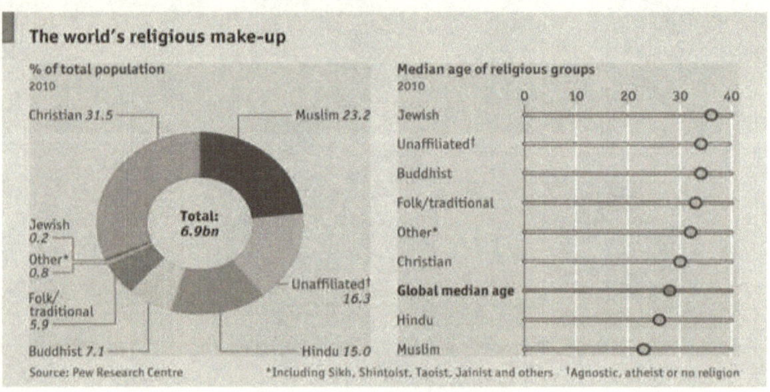

From this early indoctrination, we form our basic
constructs of what we believe is right or wrong, good or bad.
And there is nothing wrong with that. However, when we allow
our particular form of religious indoctrination to balkanize
our minds and spirits into an ⁼ us⌐ versus ⁼ them⌐
mentality, it generates unnecessary friction in social
relationships.   This phenomenon is compounded by a growing
dissatisfaction with organized religion.   While organized
religious institutions purportedly exist to bring out the
best in

humanity, historically, we. ve seen instances where
authority within religious institutions has failed their
constituents.   This is reflected in recent years in an
alarming decline in the number of people being affiliated
with an organized religious. In addition, there are so-
called Muslim extremists committing acts allegedly in the
name of Islam. These and other religious fanatics and
homicidal zealots behave in a manner which bears no
semblance to the religious doctrine upon which they claim to
be acting.   Extremism manifests itself in more way than one
way and extends well beyond Islamic extremism.

Home grown extremism across the board

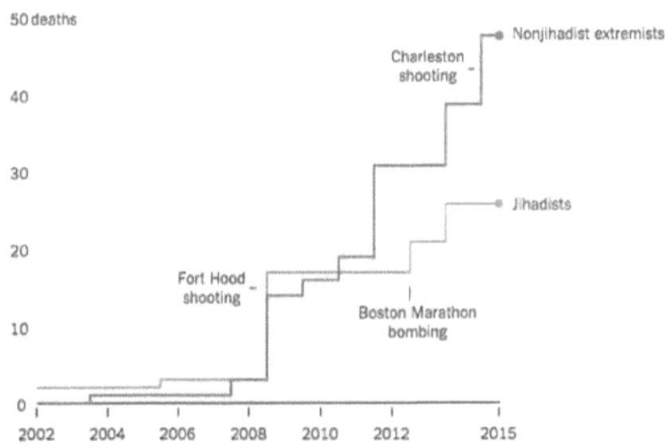

We cannot find in Scripture inflexible declarations ordering us to follow a specific religious dogma, whether it is Christianity, Islam or Judaism. In my opinion, God, Allah, Yahweh, Jehovah or related names is much less concerned about dogma and more concerned about the humanity with which we live and interact with each other.
A literal reading of the Scriptures [minus man-made interpretation/dogma] corroborates this viewpoint:

The Kingdom of Heaven is within you. Luke 17:21

Whoever purifies it [soul] has succeeded; and failure is the lot of whoever corrupts it, (Qur, an 91:9-10).

There is nothing noble in being superior to some other man. The true nobility is in being superior to your previous self. (Hindu Proverb) Guru Nanak (Sikh)

As fragrance abides in the flower, as the reflection is within the mirror, so doth thy Lord abide within thee, Why search Him without? -Prophet Mohammed (Islam)

He who knows his own self, knows God. -Yehuda Ashlag (Jewish)

35

Over time, the established religions have been perverted with an infusion of man-made concepts [inserted to facilitate political and economic domination]. These additions in a fair number of instances bear no semblance to its original teachers–Jesus, Muhammad or Moses. And historically speaking, the number of wars and conquests [3] in the name of religion, has resulted in massive losses of human life, property and dignity.

My sons. generation trend towards a new enlightenment in which spirituality versus religious dogma is where our true passion should be, despite the global eruptions of homicidal violence, disrespect of life and various extremists groups who consistently high jack religion with violence, hatred and ill-will.

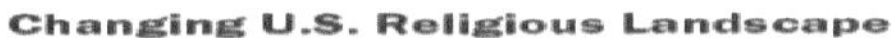

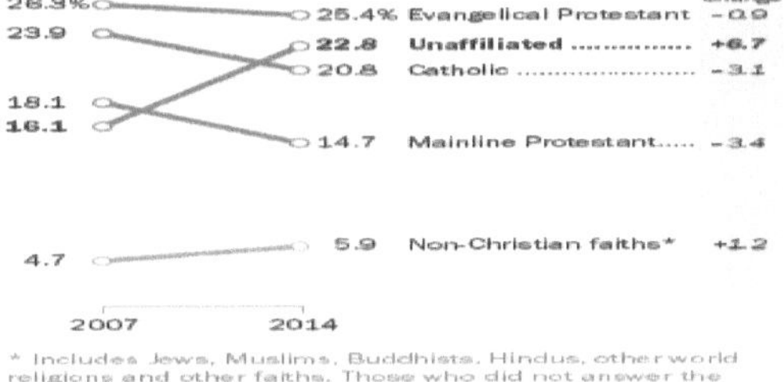

Also see Pew Research Landscape study http://www.pewforum.org/religious-landscape-study/

Our view is the principles of Islam, Christianity, Judaism, and Hinduism are all fundamentally good, but the defect is with the practitioners of these religions who don. t practice the religions they claim to follow. Ignorance is one of the greatest scourges in the world. Some Christians speak of Muslims without any knowledge of Islam, other than the small percentage of extremists who have hijacked the Islamic religion, but do not represent the principles of Islam. Some Muslims speak ill of Christians, the Holy Bible and

historical conquests without a true understanding of how
close the message of Christ and Muhammad are if you compare
the teachings.
Would it surprise us if Christians knew that Muslims view
Jesus as the Messiah?   Would it surprise us if we knew the
key figures in the Bible such as Noah, Enoch, Abraham, Moses,
David, Solomon and many others are revered in the Quran?
When people speak from ignorance, it builds artificial
divides and disseminates falsehood which then generates
negative social friction.   The more commonality we realize
exists between the various religions and " isms. [once you
remove many of the man-made, divisive elements inserted into
the various religions]; we can get to the true spirit of the
religious intent-goodness.

    The true spirit of the religion requires us to
respect Mother Earth, respect each other and fairly and
equitably interact with each other.   Once we arrive at
this place, we break down the false, dogmatic barriers and
move to a collaborative brotherhood and sisterhood that
society is in so much need.

DAD TALKS {Ignorance and religion]. Fellas, in my personal

opinion, one of the worst epidemics in society is ignorance.

I'm a big

38

proponent of robust sharing of ideas and have no problem with a differing idea as long as those in the discussion converse from a standpoint of knowledge. For instance, if we opine on a topic and have NO underlying knowledge on the specific topic (gun control, Islam, taxation, etc...), our opinion is worthless. So as we debate the social issues of the day, we should at least conduct some research on the topic before offering an opinion or just be quiet until we have learned more. People offer "expert" opinions on religion, taxation, gun control, etc... and it is obvious from their comments, these so-called "experts" have not conducted one ounce of study/research on the topic they offer opinions. We owe it to ourselves and society to become informed on whatever topic we discuss before offering "expert advice" lest we do a disservice by spreading misinformation.

As an example, homicidal, violent so-called Muslims are not representatives of the Islamic faith of over 1 billion people. I will NEVER stand for generalizing behavior of a small group of terrorists to the entire group (race, religion or otherwise). This is UNAmerican and UNconstitutional. The extremists so-called Muslims should be harshly punished and eliminated, but not the vast majority of

Muslims who reject extremism. The true Muslims should be

39

respected as believers in their faith, and partners in the
fight against terrorism.

Those within the reach of WOMP. s social media influence
know we find the best in all the religious and spiritual
teachings to bring the community together, because ⁵ it. s
not about the rightness or wrongness of our dogma, creed or
belief, it. s how we live what we claim to believe in our day
to day lives. ⁊   The Bible says, ⁵ Do unto other as you would
have other do by you⊼ (Matthew 7:12), and ⁵ love your
neighbor as you love yourself⊼ (Mark 12:31). The Quran
says, ⁵ Verily the most honored of you in the sight of Allah
is (he who is) the most righteous of you. Most honorable of
you with Allah is the one among you most careful of his/her
duty to others (Quran, Surah al-Hujurat 49:13).

My grandfather, Rev. Samuel Ross Wright, was a
Methodist minister and community activist. One of the ⁵ to
dos⊼ he assigned our church was to read the entire Bible in
one year. I undertook this challenge at age 13.
Ironically, I found a stray Bible in my Sunday school class
after Sunday school. The Bible seemed nearly new and sky
blue. I. m not sure why, but I grew attached to reading that

specific Bible. Right around the time I reached the Book of
Psalms, an older female member of the Church claimed that the
specific Bible I was reading was " her Bible" . She offered
no proof of ownership, and demanded I give " her Bible"
back? I did, but I was pretty
bummed out. In retrospect and after I completed reading the
Bible later that year, I wondered, " Why wouldn. t this elder
church member take the Bible I was reading rather than
encouraging me to read the Bible which I was doing
enthusiastically?" In a small way, this is one of the
problems of the cancerous dogma embedded within
organized religion. People under dogmatic religious remote
control get so caught up in their rituals, tithes, church
costumes, ceremonies and customs that they lose sight of the
big picture of what their religion is about: human
improvement and evolution

In reviewing some of the key Bible stories in
conversations with my sons, we always put the Bible parable
in a contemporary context to make the story RELEVANT to
today. For instance, as I. ve
mentioned in the Father-Dad chapter, my Father was not a Dad
to me. My Father was absent. However, there are key
Biblical figures where there is no " Dad " figure present.

Moses was an orphan. Regarding Jesus, Joseph is mentioned in his infancy and when Jesus

41

was 12 year old at the Temple, but you never read of
Joseph. s presence with Jesus after that. Jesus is more
closely aligned with his mother, Mary.

The Prophet of Islam, Muhammad, was born in the year 570
in the town of Mecca, a mountain town in the high desert
plateau of western Arabia. His name derives from the Arabic
verb hamada, meaning "to praise, to glorify." He was the
first and only son of Abd Allah bin Al-Muttalib and Amina
bint Wahb. Abd Allah died before Muhammad's birth and
Muhammad was raised by his mother
Amina. When Muhammad was five or six his mother took him to
Yathrib, an oasis town a few hundred miles north of Mecca, to
stay with relatives and visit his father's grave there. On
the return journey, Amina took ill and died. Muhammad was an
orphan.

From these stories, I drew strength knowing that
inspired individuals, having a profound impact on history,
shared something in common with me. When my sons asked about
my father, without excusing my father. s irresponsible
behavior, I always used these stories to explain that the
Universe had a greater purpose for me in NOT having my Father
in my life than having him in my life. This is

what religion that fuels spirituality does. It empowers us
to see our lives and challenges through stories of a person
or group of people who overcame the same challenge. And
this gives us hope and strength to do the same in our own
lives.

Summary

Surely, the Kingdom of Heaven is within us. The
carbon, nitrogen and oxygen atoms in our bodies, as well as,
atoms of all other heavy elements were created in previous
generations of
stars over 4.5 billion years ago. Because humans and every
other animal, as well as, most of the matter on Earth
contain these
elements, we are literally made of the Universe. s material.
So the statement the ʺ kingdom of heaven is within us, is
true on both the spiritual and physical realm when you
factor in the materials from the Universe-an invisible
power- that comprise our bodies. And the existence of this
invisible power, which science calls ʺ Dark Matter and Dark
Energy, (95 percent of matter) that impacts and influences
the expansion of the Universe, is real. Even though neither

Dark Matter nor Dark Energy can be seen with the naked eye
does not

43

mean it is non-existent. (See NASA:

http://science.nasa.gov/astrophysics/focus-areas/what-is-dark-energy/)

   It is perfectly normal to explore religion or not explore religion. It is also okay for us to accept a particular religion, which may be best suited for our soul. s advancement and evolution. However, the acceptance of another religion by someone else doesn. t mean that person is not going to heaven nor does it mean this is a bad person. It simply means they have found a different path to hopefully the same destination, peace and contentment. Moreover, some will reject religion altogether, yet have developed their own brand of ethics and spirituality to guide them through life. Our message is simple, if we are in a dark room; we need as many candles as possible to provide light. As long as whatever we practice brings forth that light, it should be respected, accepted and understood.

   Finally, I am a believer in God. My belief in the power of God has served as the foundation of my entire existence, evolution and success. My relationship to God with my own personal failings and stumbles is best summarized in the words of Denzel Washington [whose father was a Pentecostal minister for 50 years] when he was quoted as follows:

*" Put God first in everything you do ⋯
Everything that I have is by the grace of
God,
understand that. It's a gift ⋯ I didn't
always
stick with Him, but He stuck with me. "* —
Denzel Washington to College Grads:　"Put
God First in Everything You Do〟,
Relevant
Magazine, May 11, 2015

<u>CHAPTER 3:   SIMPLE LIVING</u> :

*Man. Because he sacrifices his health in order to make money.
Then he sacrifices money to recuperate his health. And then he
is so
anxious about the future that he does not enjoy the present;
the result being that he does not live in the present or the
future; he lives as if he is never going to die, and then dies
having never really lived.*

-Dalai Lama

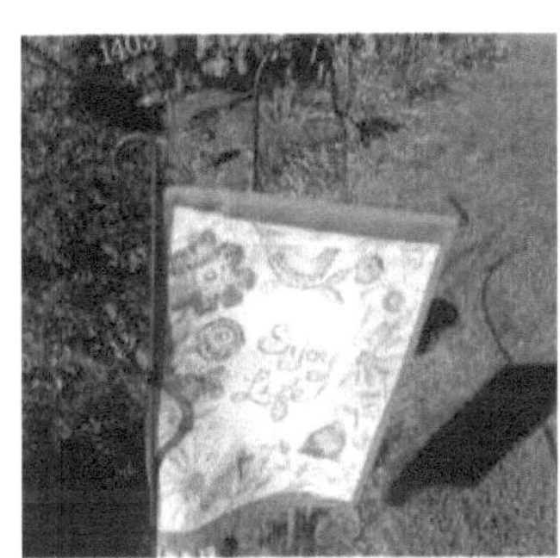

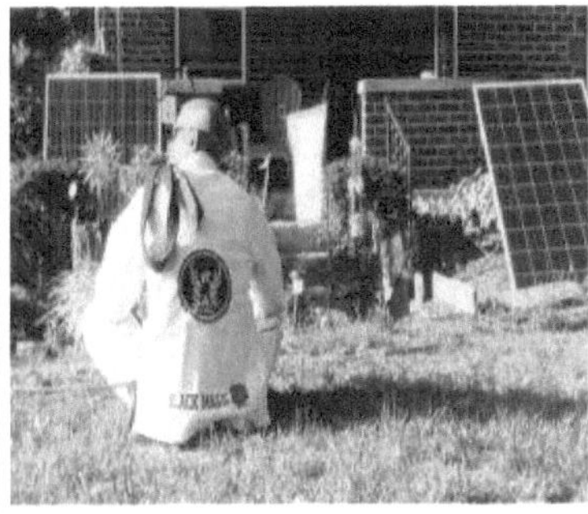

Basking in the Sun

<u>Dad Talks</u> [Alone time]. My sons asked me: "Why have you over the

years gotten up so early on weekday and some weekend mornings

(5:30-5:45 AM)?" Me: "Because I like to kiss the Sun when it rises, get

my blood flowing, get to know myself, and wake up with the Earth to

46

align my day with the increases and decreases in
sunlight/Circadian rhythms. I make a conscious effort to
align my lifestyle to nature for good flow." A good day
begins with a connection to the Universe, meditation,
cleansing, exercise and focus for that day. s tasks. There a
few key areas to be discussed that clash with the idea of
Simple Living: financial insecurity, interpersonal
relationships and attitude. This quote from Harvard Business
Review ("Executives, Protect Your Alone Time", December 16,
2015) hits the nail on the head:

*In our contemporary offices and always-busy
lives, alone time can be difficult to come by. But
successful creative thinkers share a need for
solitude. They make a practice of turning away
from the distractions of daily life to give their
minds space to reflect, make new connections, and
find meaning.*

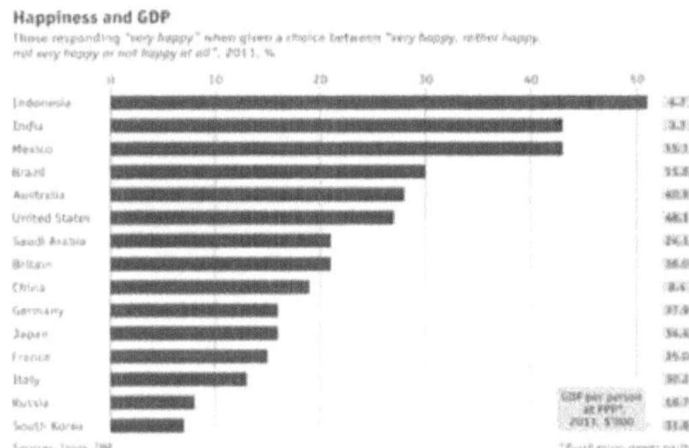

Financial insecurity

If our lifestyle has us on the eternal treadmill of endless
desires and living above our means, then we. re already
living a non-simple life. Our ability to participate in
meaningful life reflection is stilted.

It. s stilted because our mind is constantly bombarded with
how we will pay for this, that or the other, some of which we
don. t need in the first place. We need to step back,
carefully analyze how we got to this state of being, and what
we can do to escape from it? If we continue in this state
of insecurity, our meditative abilities and
spiritual growth discussed in Chapter 2, and then we will not
reach our full potential. There are many financial decisions
in life we can transact more intelligently.

Should we really buy a new car or could we get a less
expensive used car to reduce our monthly car note?
Do we really need a SUV that could transport an
aircraft carrier or a less gas consuming vehicle?
Do we really need a house that has excessive amounts of
living space when a house half the size could meet our
needs?
Do we need 100 channels via cable TV paying over $100
per month and billed as if we watch TV 24X7 when we
could buy a streaming device to watch TV on demand, add
a few pay channels and save half the money we spend?
How much discretionary spending is done on high
interest (high cost to borrow money) credit cards when
we could intelligently wait or purchase the items same
as cash without interest?

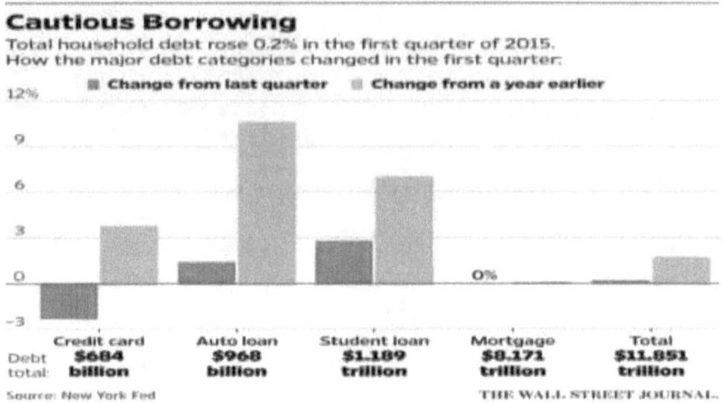

Astronomical consumer debt

This list of self-generated financial stress could go on and on, but the point is we should temper our desires to match what we truly need, which leads us into the next topic: debt. We go into debt when we don. t have enough money in our pockets, bank accounts or other liquid resources to purchase the items we want with cash. However, when you borrow money from someone, a bank or your friend, you are partially under that person. s control, because you create a legal commitment to pay the money back to that person or bank. This creates additional stress. The debt also comes with an interest charge, which is a fancy word for the cost we pay to borrow the money. If you loan me $100 with 10 percent annual interest, then I

must pay you back $110. The $10 is the cost you assess me to
borrow the money. Some people will never pay back the actual
principal ($100) debt they owe but just the minimum interest
payment

[especially on consumer credit cards]. Both poor people and
more income producing people fall into this same trap. Many
professional people with high incomes are as broke as the
poor person. It. s just a matter of scale. Whether high
income generators or not, if you only pay back the finance/
interest charge, you stay on the eternal debt treadmill,
which means you are in a constant state of high stress.
And God forbid you don. t pay back the debt at all, because
that person or bank can take you to court, obtain a judgment
against you and start taking things that belong to you, such
as your pay check, house, and bank account and then report
you as a bad credit risk to Equifax, Transunion and Experion.
And this makes it costlier for you to borrow in the future
for the next seven years.

   Now, there is good debt if borrowed in reasonable
amounts for items we can afford such as:

   1. Home loan

   2. Reasonable educational

loans

3. Reasonable business loans

4. Reasonable, calculated investments (stock &
bond combos established companies)

5. Balance transfers/same as cash transactions
as long   as you pay off before interests kicks
in and no additions to existing debt

<u>DAD Talks.</u> [Don. t add stress to your life unnecessarily].
Fellas, much of the stress and anxiety we suffer from are
based upon the excessive complication we knowingly and
willingly inject into our lives. We then complain about the
very thing we voluntarily granted safe passage into our
lives. Eliminate *complification* !

<u>DAD Talks</u> (Finance stress abatement with finance and
contentment):

    1. <u>INVESTING:</u> Fellas if you have a safe,
decent,   operable car that you own (which you
do), it   would be smarter to put $200-500 per
month   in stocks/mutual funds v. a new car or any
    asset which depreciates substantially.
Why?

    Assets which depreciate immediately and

continue to depreciate give you nothing
back v. a good stocks/mutual funds will
grow your $200-500 per month as long as
you pick the right investments (and that's
where I come in).
To make the math simple, if you assume a
10% return and $400 monthly investment
(v.
car payment), you can earn nearly $500
annual investment return and that's
without
compounding. The choice is yours.

2. . <u>ESTATE PLANNING</u>: Fellas, when I
transition unless you conduct yourselves
like complete fools, you.11 have
financial stability.
I've scanned and emailed to you all the
relevant account summary info for all
investment, retirement, bank and life
insurance accounts, etc...so if I go, you
know EXACTLY what to do. There is nothing
worse than scrambling around trying to
figure out where important documents are

while your grieving loss. Do the same

thing if you have

53

children. By the way, the money will go
to a
trust (managed by a financial
institution) and
you will NOT have access to the principal
until age 30.
3. CORE BELIEFS: In a contest between
being liked/accepted in this world and
your core beliefs, ALWAYS opt for your
core beliefs, because even though someone
may not
like/accept you, they will respect you.
And I'd much rather have respect than to
be
liked/accepted or have to be a social
chameleon changing my core beliefs with
each social circumstance. I recommend you
conduct yourselves the same way.

Interpersonal relationships

Interpersonal relationships are essential to life
satisfaction. We can have all the money we think we want
and yet be extremely unhappy and life dissatisfied. Our

relationships with key people-family and close friends-gives
us a sense of connectedness to something bigger

54

than ourselves.   While we all need solitude for self
reflection and growth, sustained and unbalanced aloneness is
counter productive to human advancement on a individual or
group basis.   Angus Chen, NPR writer, wrote about
"loneliness":

*Loneliness has been linked to everything from heart
disease to Alzheimer's disease. Depression is common
among the lonely. Cancers tear through their bodies
more rapidly, and viruses hit them harder and more
frequently. In the short term, it feels like the loneliness
will kill you. A study suggests that's because the pain of
loneliness activates the immune pattern of a primordial
response commonly known as fight or flight.* (NPR,
"Loneliness May Warp Our Genes, And Our
Immune Systems", November 29, 2015)

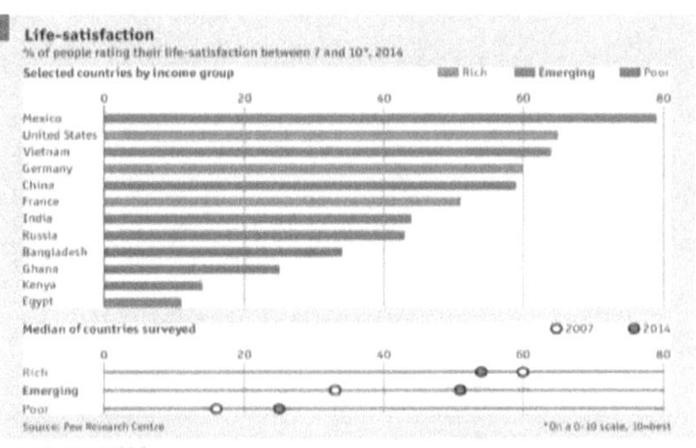

This chart shows that citizens of countries in emerging
markets are within a whisker of expressing the same level
of satisfaction with their lives as people in rich
countries.   They are as happy with less material stuff.

    Positive interpersonal connections start with our own families.
I think of my own rearing and family connection and how that
influenced my development as a human being.   And this
doesn. t mean that you have to have 24 X 7 contact with
everyone in your family.   But it does mean we have
meaningful and honest
engagement when we do connect, especially in our formative
years.
There will be people in our families we don. t get along
with as in regular society. There is no need to fake the
funk on that reality. We

should perhaps give that family person greater latitude since they are blood relatives, but most of the prophets in the Bible found their closest allies and followers with non-blood related associates. None of Jesus. disciples were from his immediate or extended family.

Nevertheless, embrace and stayed connected with your family.

Family bonds and connection is crucial to a solid foundation whether that family is by blood, adoption or close association. It also means that within our families we have a strongest, consistent connection with those in our immediate circle. Fortifying those relationships means we eat one meal together each day. It means we have actual voice and in-person contact versus text only. It means we spend time in conversation talking about life-problems, goals, disappointments. The same principles hold true for friends. We must reach out and talk to our friends without needing or wanting anything from them. How. s it going? We must take a personal interest in things that they are doing or struggling with. In the past year, I. ve had two people I knew who took their own life because they lost hope. Suicide became their only perceived option, because they lacked a strong interpersonal

connection and had reached the lowest point of life
satisfaction.

57

We must not allow this to happen to each other. The
interpersonal relationships we forge help us, as well as,
help the people we reach out to connect.

<u>Attitude</u>

Finally, our attitude about our life experience forms
a critical basis for life satisfaction and simple living.
There will be highs and lows in our personal and
professional worlds.

In September 2015, I competed for the first time as a
Brazilian Jiu Jitsu black belt in Las Vegas as the Masters
World
Championships. The prior year, I won the gold medal as a
brown belt. I trained as hard for the black belt competition
as I had done for the brown belt competition, but I came up
short in the black belt division, losing a decision in the
quarter finals. I was disappointed in the result, but I knew
within my heart I had trained hard and given my best. The
referee, after neither of us scored any points or
advantages against each other, awarded the match to my
opponent. I shook the referee and my opponent. s hand. I
huddled with team, but then I moved on chalking it up to a
learning experience.

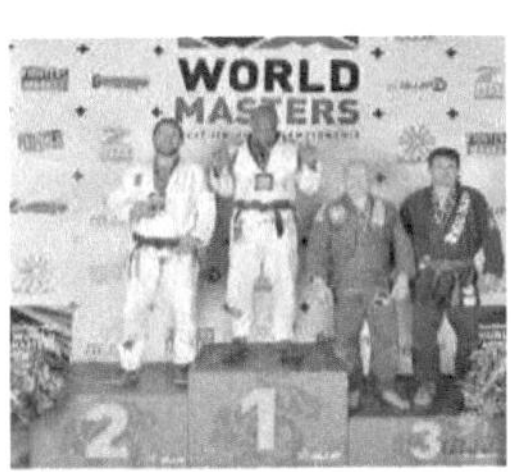

Brown belt
  victory

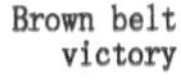
Long Beach, CA,

v.

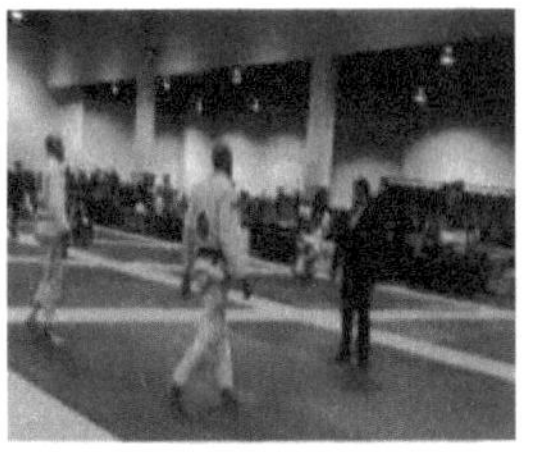

Black belt defeat

(Las Vegas

DAD Talk: {Accept adversity and roll through it]. So
I've gotten this question one or two times, "Do you ever get
down, you always seem so happy?" Me: "Thank you. I am
happy. I don't get "down" as you put it, because I've
accepted adversity as a part of life itself-death, periodic
financial struggles, professional and personal challenges
which last for a season. The acceptance of adversity builds a
solution oriented mindset to face whatever the adversity is
to overcome it, rather than to resist what is a part of life,
or ignore it as if it will not happen. However, over time, we
should have accumulated enough life wisdom through prior
adversity to sidestep potential future adversity/stress
without walking into it, thereby creating more
stress/anxiety. This perspective on life enhances our
happiness,

because we have imposed less unnecessary stress on our lives. Bottom line: Our attitude should be to accept and roll with the adversity we face, and DON'T overcommit to non-core, discretionary life obligations, because that produces self-created unnecessary stress, and anxiety that we then complain about to the world. Saying "No" [not just to drugs] is a beautiful thing. The use of " no" can be a very liberating experience, and reduces our anxiety.

Summary

As much as we try to make personal finance unmanageable and stressful, personal finance is really just applying simple mathematics we learned in elementary school. If you know how to read, and perform basic addition and subtraction, then you are automatically empowered to save for a house, start a business, invest and plan for retirement. So please do the following:

1. Spend less than you earn;
2. Earn more: Second or third job, go back to school for training, start a side business
3. Live frugal (which does not mean be cheap): wisely allocate resources, delay purchases, coupon

4. Manage Money: open checking/savings account develop a plan to pay off debt, starting with the highest interest rate debt, invest in a 401(k)/403, Roth IRA, regular IRA; you don. t need a million to do this. Start smart and make steady

contributions

5. Budget: create specific goals with specific numbers for major expenses like home, vacation, and longer goals including college savings (if applicable) and retirement

Interpersonal relationships are required to help reach our goals in life. We can. t do it alone. We must make a concentrated effort to create and sustain meaningful relationships with friends and family.
These connections and the positive friction from these connections refine and uplift us as human beings.

Attitude determines altitude. We have to face and overcome adversity, strive and struggle. When you think about the process for how a diamond is produced, there is wisdom in the process. A diamond is rock subject to massive amounts of pressure and heat to become an unbreakable mineral. We become diamonds in life only if we have the courage and temerity to withstand the heat and pressure

61

of living. Attitude is what determines if we have the
ability to withstand it. We must attitudinally behave like
the palm tree, pliable and yet firm when needed to adapt and
ultimately overcome
difficulty.

<u>CHAPTER 4: WELLNESS: NUTRITION + FITNESS</u>

" You are what you eat! " - Anonymous

<u>Nutrition</u>

For some reason, nutrition has been turned into a
mystical art that only the high priests of the Shaolin Temple
of Nutrition can unlock and figure out. There is the Paleo
diet, the Atkins diet, the South Beach diet and any number of
diets all designed to give us optimal health. Rather than
bang our heads against the wall trying to sort through every
diet on the market, we should simply examine the essential
needs of the human body. In the final analysis, we need
portioned amounts of protein, complex carbohydrates, simple
carbohydrates, and water.

Unfortunately, our society has turned to magic pills,
diets and " Messianic" , quick fix exercise plans that will
supposedly give us the physique of an Olympian. This is
fantasy nutritional foolishness, which will NOT work.
Vitamin and other supplements are just that, " supplements" .
This means the core (non-supplement) nutrition we

need must come from the foods we eat.   Because of the

astronomical growth in laziness and quick fixes instead of

accepting that nutrition and fitness requires active,

consistent participation, we look for short cuts (surgeries,

dangerous supplements, steroids).

     Rather than mislead people as if Wright On My People

has the secret nutrition formula, it is recommended that you

consume food with the ranges of the " well balanced diet"

depicted below. Also, there are numerous free web sites

which will create a nutrition plan for you. You only have

to input certain nutrition goals and it will generate the

plan. Now, it is still up to us to follow the plan, and

prepare the food to consume. A computer, a trainer, a

pimped out kitchen, thousands of recipes books and related

helpful guides cannot do the work. You have to do the work!

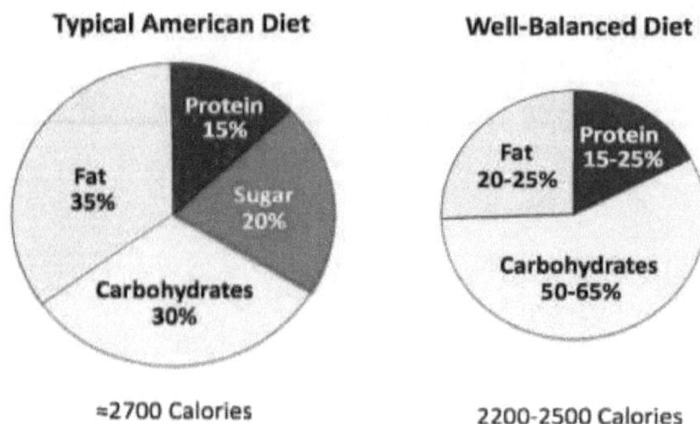

Nutrition empowerment: Create your own nutrition plan:

https://www.eatthismuch.com/

In my opinion, the manner in which you consume your complex and simple carbohydrates, protein and good fats is your choice. Some people eat pork, others do not. Some are vegans, others eat meat. Again, whatever you chose in terms of specific foods, you can go to the free web site above. Based upon your weight, nutrition goals and activity level you determine your nutrition needs. The biggest thing to remember is that a pill, supplement, magic fruit potion or related mystical juice will not get you to where you want to be.

How to Spot Malnutrition	And How to Remedy It
The presence of two or more of these factors indicates that a patient is malnourished, according to guidelines from nutrition and dietetic societies:	These are some of the things you can do at home, even if you don't feel hungry, to help ensure you get the nourishment your body needs.
• Insufficient food intake compared with nutrition requirements	• Eat five or six small meals a day
• Weight loss over time	• Eat a bigger meal earlier in the day
• Loss of muscle mass	• Have easy, convenient meals and nutritious snacks on hand
• Loss of fat mass	• Eat nutrient-rich foods, such as low-fat yogurt, cheese, and nuts
• Fluid accumulation	
• Measurably diminished grip strength	• Prepare and freeze extra servings

The Affordable Care Act was passed and signed into law in the United States and many state governments have in some cases separate and in other cases complimentary health care laws on the books to promote improvements in global health. Without meandering through the political landmines pertaining to health care, the reality is many citizens of many nations are severely challenged with health concerns, some of which are directly traced to insufficient nutrition. The latest media emphasis has been on obesity. The number of overweight people in the US has grown significantly.

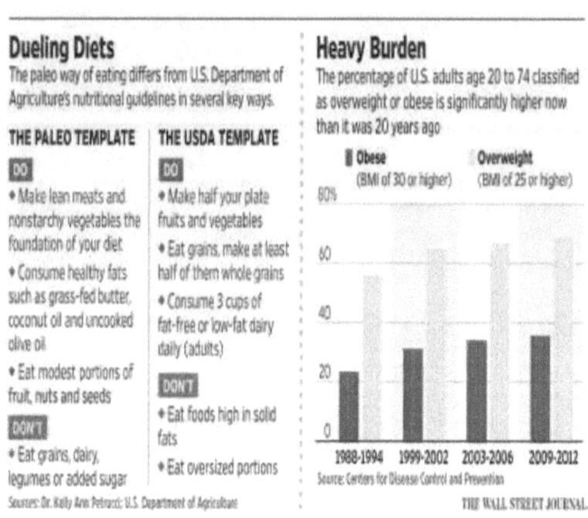

Dueling Diets

The paleo way of eating differs from U.S. Department of Agriculture's nutritional guidelines in several key ways.

THE PALEO TEMPLATE

DO
- Make lean meats and nonstarchy vegetables the foundation of your diet
- Consume healthy fats such as grass-fed butter, coconut oil and uncooked olive oil
- Eat modest portions of fruit, nuts and seeds

DON'T
- Eat grains, dairy, legumes or added sugar

THE USDA TEMPLATE

DO
- Make half your plate fruits and vegetables
- Eat grains, make at least half of them whole grains
- Consume 3 cups of fat-free or low-fat dairy daily (adults)

DON'T
- Eat foods high in solid fats
- Eat oversized portions

Sources: Dr. Kelly Ann Petrucci; U.S. Department of Agriculture

Heavy Burden

The percentage of U.S. adults age 20 to 74 classified as overweight or obese is significantly higher now than it was 20 years ago

Obese (BMI of 30 or higher) / Overweight (BMI of 25 or higher)

1988-1994, 1999-2002, 2003-2006, 2009-2012

Source: Centers for Disease Control and Prevention

THE WALL STREET JOURNAL.

I prepare and consume five or six smaller portioned controlled meals per day and I eat a junk snack on Friday evening. We have to own our nutrition, which may requires us to take time away from watching TV, doodling on the computer, talking on the phone or some other useless, mindless activity for an hour to plan and cook our nutrition. It is our job to spend more time owning our health. It is not your doctor. s sole responsibility. It is your duty as a human being.

<u>Fitness</u>

There is an intensified focus on health globally, especially fitness. We are bombarded with TV commercials, promotions, video clips and advice on how to be fit.   In concert with the section on nutrition, a solid fitness plan must be created. Each person has to develop their own flow on how they prefer to exercise (alone v. group), what exercises to do (weight, yoga, swimming, biking, etc···) when to exercise (AM or PM) and how frequently to exercise per week. In my opinion, as long as, you get the exercise consistent with your fitness goals, and work the required muscles with cardio, then all of the exercise specifics, similar to nutrition, should be determined by each person.

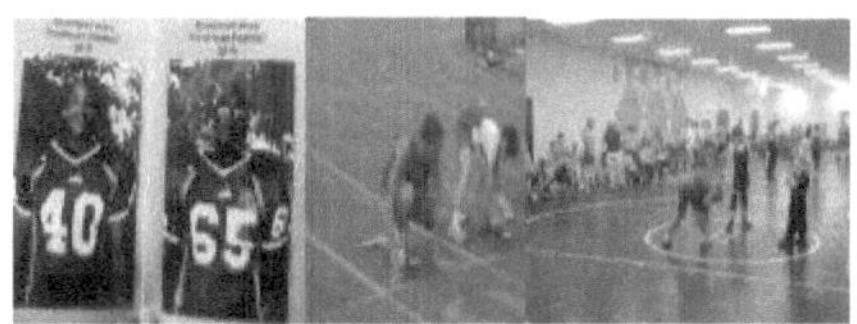

Like nutrition, far too many people are seeking a fitness savior, who will just about do everything for us. If we desire to be

fit, we have to have the focus, discipline and commitment to do it. A trainer, coach or partner in group exercise can.t do the exercises for you. You have to do it, even on days when you are not as motivated.

I. m not a proponent of telling people what do to, but I will share with you what I do.   I exercise six days a week, combining Brazilian Jiu Jitsu, plyometric, biking, cardio machines, yoga,
weights, core and other exercises to build an athletic body. That is my goal. My nutrition intake of protein is about 1.7 times my lean body weight. I wake up every weekday around 5:30 AM. I drink 12 oz. of water mixed with apple cider vinegar and lemon. I then drink a 12 oz. packet of aspartame-free energy (caffeine) power (10 packets from Kroger less than $ 2 per packet). I then do 30-35 minutes of cardio, lower/upper abdominal/core exercises, and eight sets of strength exercises focused on various muscles in the body. I rotate muscles groups from day to day with weight/strength training. Now what I do is not necessarily what anyone else should do. Over years of experimentation, I. ve found the proper balance I desire that meets my goals in terms of body build and health overall.

).

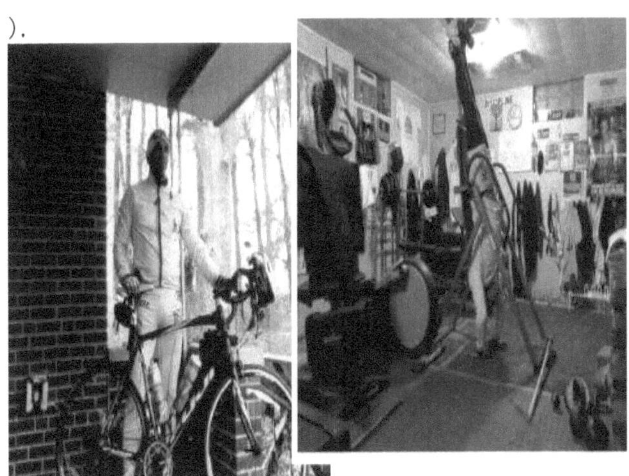

Here is a basic chart of some suggested fitness activities:

    I often joke in social media discourse about the difficulty I have in maintaining my fitness regimen in the winter months
(December, January and February).   I. m an early morning exercise 70

person with a 5:30 AM wake up time on weekdays.   The
combination of increased darkness, cold temperatures and
reduced Vitamin D can stunt motivation and desire. I
collectively refer to this phenomenon as the ᵗ Sleep
Gorilla꞉ -darkness, cold and Vitamin D deficiency. To
overcome the Sleep Gorilla, I. ll go to bed earlier, use a
wake up light in our bedroom to artificially mimic the
gradual increase of Sunlight in warmer months, and take
Vitamin D

supplements.   We have to make small tweaks to our
environment, as well as, to increase our probability of
reaching our fitness goals and having the body we desire.

Summary

There are no magical nutrition and fitness solutions.
We recommend eating a portioned based clean nutrition plan.
It is okay to drink alcohol -though I. m not much of an
alcohol drinker-and eat some junk in moderation [not
multiple times per day, perhaps once per week].   The sooner
society a stop looking for magic dust and quick fixes to
nutrition and fitness, the better off we are.

I. ve come to conclusion that many people know the
basics of both fitness and nutrition. They have access to
a gym membership

71

and/or exercise equipment. However, they lack the discipline
and motivation to act on what they know. No one can give
that to us, not a trainer or coach. From our discussion on
Spirituality in Chapter 2, discipline and motivation MUST
also come from within.

CHAPTER 5 :   LIFE SUCCESS

What is success? Life success is a very personal
journey that we all have to define for ourselves. Of course,
in order to achieve life success, we must comply with the
basic law of the land, and behave toward our fellow human
being with dignity and respect.

Success is not material wealth, a specific plateau, or
achievement. Success represents a combination of variables
that drive and motivate future positive behavior. In high-
school, there is always those infamous awards including,
" The Person Most Likely to Succeed" . From our perspective,
the person most likely to succeed is the person who brings
the proper level of introspection, focus,
discipline, motivation, and compassion to their lives. And
this
person will never quit in the pursuit of their goals. All of
us have the inherent potential to be " the most likely person
to succeed" ; however, we have an increasing number of people
who settle for mediocrity. And another segment of our
population not succeeding are terrified of failure, so these
folks rarely put themselves at any level of
vulnerability due to the fear of NOT succeeding.

DAD TALKS: What if I told you that
people and being in the land of unhappiness is traced to
their failure to conduct a brutally honest self-assessment?
Some people go their entire lifetimes without conducting a
self-assessment, and these people tend to be unhappy and
unsuccessful. The failure to conduct this self-assessment,
which has to be ongoing as opposed to a one-time event,
results in aimlessly jumping from one thing, person and
interest to the next in an attempt to find happiness and
success externally through that thing, person or interest.
When we discover we aren't successful, then confusion,
boredom and dissatisfaction set in and then off we float to
the next best thing once again seeking "happiness" and
success. And this cycle continues over and over and over.
Success and happiness begins with assessing those peculiar,
unique internal factors we all have and matching those
factors to how we live our lives, how we interact with other
people, what job or career we select, and reflecting those
success factors in our
associations, interests and goals.

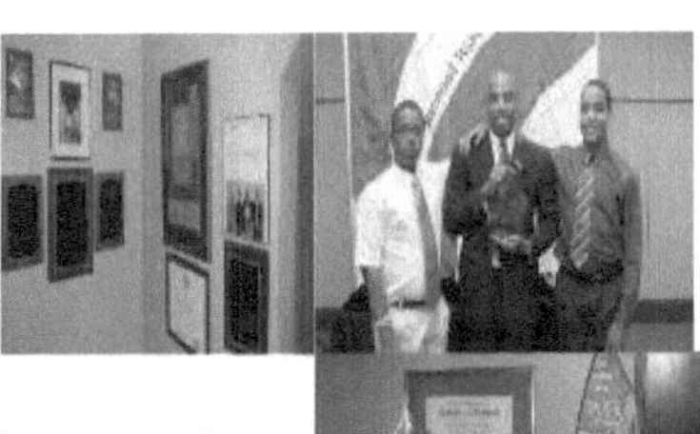

Professional, community service and martial arts awards

For us, success starts with a self-assessment and
understanding our purpose based upon these two fundamental
questions:

Why are we here?
What gifts or natural talents do we have to reach
our full potential and help others?

The answer to these two questions is obtained only after
critical introspection, and feedback from those in our
immediate circle. We should recruit a few people to be on
our informal board of directors to give us honest feedback
and guidance for our lives. This board should be folks we
trust, respect and who have a track record of success in
their lives.

Here was the methodology I used to find my purpose and
assist my children with finding their purpose.   Growing

up, I was analytical, decent at math and loved to read. I

enjoyed science,

75

especially the weather and astronomy. I was also very verbal and loved good discussions of many topics. My family was very vocal and our family reunions were and still are lively events infused with fun, and political/social debates. When I was deciding what my purpose was, I asked myself what these skills can be used for in the real world. For a short time, I was going to be a meteorologist, then a minister and then I decided after I started watching the CNN Show " Crossfire‚ in my senior year of high-school debates on law as a career. I started following political and social news and decided that I should be a lawyer.

When I entered college, I entered with the idea that I was going to law school, so I needed to get really good grades and stay socially and politically active to sharpen my negotiation, analytical and debating skills. After over 20 years of actively practicing law with two large global companies (still employed at one), a law firm, the prosecutor‚ s office and teaching at two universities, I made the right choice. I love what I can do with my law degree for myself and for others. But the right choice for me began with me discussing my purpose, assessing my skill set and matching it to a career. Success in my career came naturally because I intrinsically liked what I did, and

continue to like what I do. I discovered my purposeand
acted to obtain the educational training to succeed at my
profession. Success for me was contentment, financial
earning capacity to support my family and various causes,
influencing society through volunteer service, help people
who had legal needs, earning respect from my peers and
leaving a robust legacy to pass on to my sons.

My sons are in this same ³ life success₨ process now.
At their high-school, the guidance counselor offered for both
my sons to do a career assessment. These self-assessments
consisted of a
questionnaire they completed to articulate their interests, a
questionnaire to the parents, feedback from their teachers
and their academic performance in school. All of these data
points were integrated and then formulated to create a career
profile of what professions match up with my sons. intrinsic
interest.   Malachi leaned more artistic with computer flair
so right now his focus is Digital Arts Design and Electronic
Media. On the other hand, Bilal. s interest revolved around
robotics, engineering and cartography. Once we had this data,
we had an idea of where their career interests should be
channeled.

The next item we had to clear is that there was a market for these skills and the specific professions. There was. Finally, we analyzed what type of training or education is needed for them to do that profession. Is a master. s degree, bachelor. s degree, or associate. s degree needed or none at all? We figured out what was required and they enrolled in programs after high-school to start on the path to fulfill their purpose.

In addition to the career self-assessment, I. d periodically ask my sons, why do you think you are here on Earth?   I know that sounds like a heavy question, but I wanted their brains to process and think over that. I was less concerned with a ⁵ correct͙ answer and more interested in sparking my sons to be introspective. Their answers were what you would expect between the ages of 12-20 years old. There was uncertainty, but a basic comfort level that the professional options before them matched up with what they thought they should be doing in life.

I decided sharing my story and that of my own children would be much more connective to the reading audience, providing
intimate and useful knowledge rather than pontificating about

professional success in a vacuum. My sons continue to
pursue their professional goals. The beginning of the
process began in 10th grade, not halfway through their first
year of college on a whim. The problem in our society today
is we see children going to college having no clue
whatsoever what their purpose and interests are.
They. ve done no introspection to determine that. It is our
job as parents to help our children with this based upon the
life wisdom we hopefully have by the time our own children
are about to start their own careers.   There may still have
to be modifications and
adjustments as they travel their path, but at least they
start with a basic roadmap to increase the probability of
success.

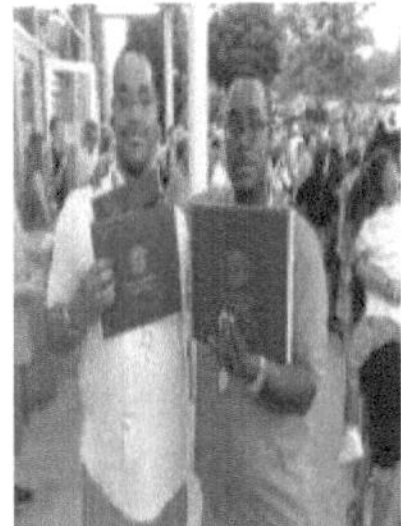 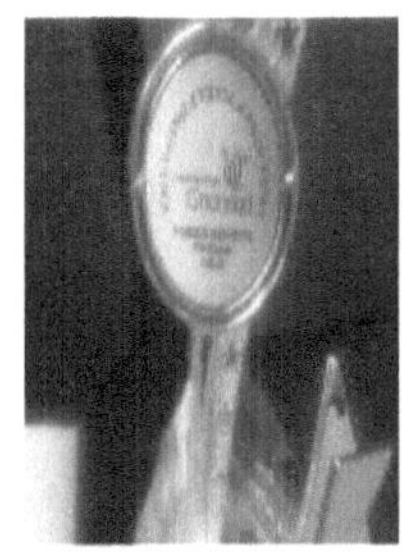 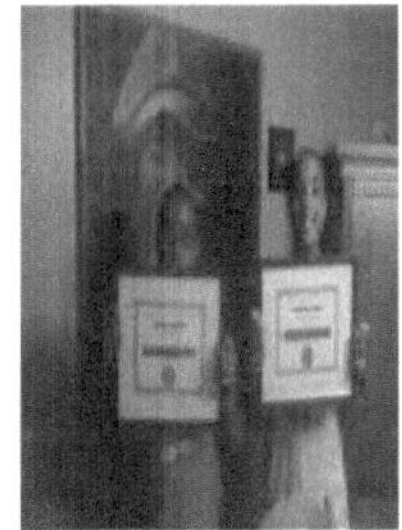

Educational success

In the Father-Dad Chapter, we discussed the importance
of time accountability for the time we allocate to various
daily activities having 168 hours available in a week. In the
final analysis, even using the most liberal allocations of
time, there are anywhere from 12-15 hours per week of
"missing time" in most people's schedules if they are
brutally honest with time accounting.

If we take the average of this " missing time"
calculation (13.5 hours=810 minutes), we discover there is
ample time available to do most of what we need to do to
achieve whatever we define as our personal success (exercise
more, read a book, household projects, church attendance,
start a small business, school work, family time, volunteer
work, etc...) The question is what is being done with the
lost or "missing time" in our schedule now? Where is it?
Perform an audit of your own time allocations, minute by
minute and modify your schedule to align with life success.

People assert, "I don't have enough time to do X", or
achieve sub-par/mediocre success in life overall due to the
"I have no time" excuse. In many instances, this happens
because they lack the ability to prioritize their core
activities from " most important" to " least

important, have very disorganized/jumbled operating principles of living, and in some cases are just down, right lazy.

A pre-requisite for success in life is knowing how we allocate our time right now. Once there is specific time accountability into what we are doing, we will discover ample opportunities to re-direct the bulk of our time to those items we have prioritized as most important. When we do this, we attain greater success in life.

GIVING BACK AND HELPING OTHERS

" To whom much is given, much is required, (Luke 12:48). Jesus, speaking to the people, once said, " The harvest is great, but the laborers are few. " (Matt 9:37). There are similar exhortations found in the Quran, Bhagavad Gita, Talmud and related religious/spiritual texts. Our view of success incorporates the idea that we must contribute to the advancement of others without any expectation of reward or financial compensation. We do it, because it is the right thing to do.

As Wright On My People drives positive social change, we are most proud of the fact that none of our principles were compromised in our journey striving for life success, which

lasts a lifetime. We

81

never had to rob, cheat, steal or exploit anyone to get
what we wanted. In fact, we. ve taken quite the opposite
road with volunteer service to the Freestore Foodbank,
Salvation Army, Christmas and Thanksgiving soup kitchens
and gift giving drives, scholarship fundraisers, and
service on various community boards. Our
philosophy is, if we live our lives with a closed fist, no
one can take anything away from us, but we will not receive
any blessings from the Universe. So it is much better to
live our life with an open hand than a closed fist, because
we will be more blessed to receive in abundance.

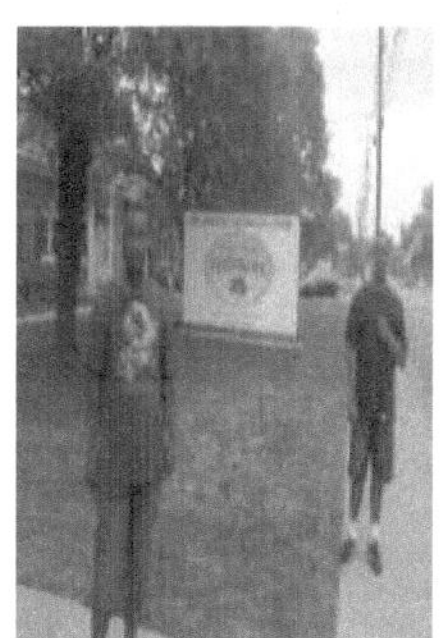
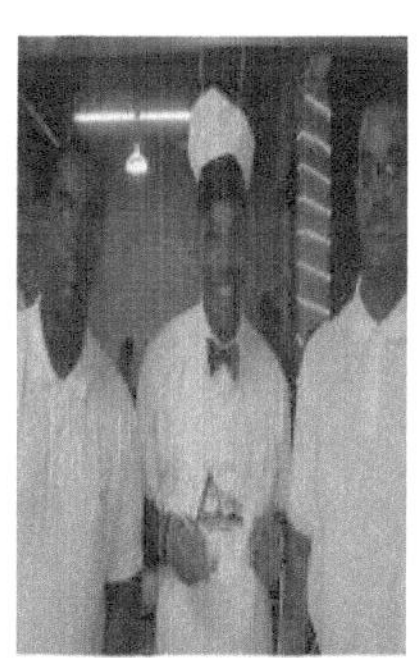
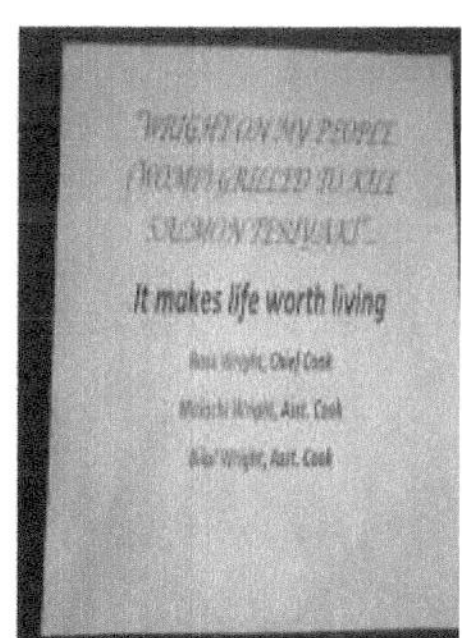

Volunteers: Freestore Foodbank and " Men Who Love Cooking" scholarship
fundraiser

"No person is an island unto themselves."   Whether
we want to admit it or not, there is a universal social
connectedness we have to each other as human beings. I
consider myself a very independent person all the way down to
installing solar panels to supply a large portion of our
household electricity needs, as well as, raising chickens for
food, cultivating a garden to grow vegetables, storing months
worth of dry food, and storing other items to sustain
ourselves in the event of some societal calamity
independently. Notwithstanding our fierce independence, we
need each other.

Leveraging the concepts we discussed about time
accountability in the previous chapter, we have plenty time
to help others. We should never leave helping other citizens
solely to
somebody else. And the helping doesn't require us to create
a tax-exempt foundation, write a million dollar check or give
a body organ, though it could be these things as well. The
simple things people need in society everyday we can all chip
in to help in those areas. We can all allocate a few hours
per month to whtaever charity,
organization or group that is involved in these efforts to

make a difference in someone. s life. So as the Nike

commercial advises, " Just Do It ! .

83

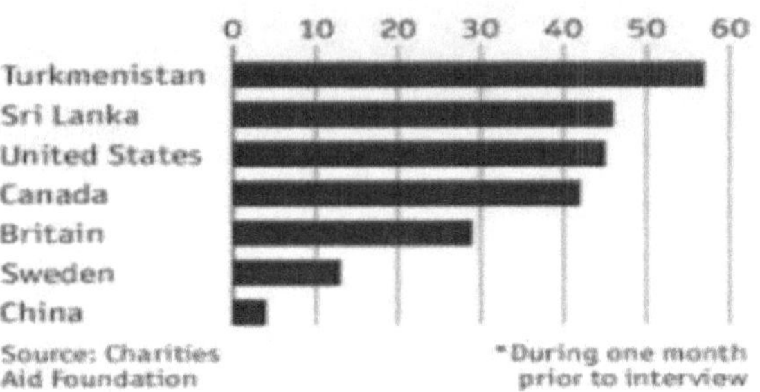

Economists 2013

And for those of us who may be more affluent, we can contribute to organizations with 501(c) (3) tax exempt status to get a tax break while giving at the same time. We. ve donated hundreds of dollars in items which are stil usable to the Salvation Army and elsewhere to a person or family who can use the item (computers, exercise equipment, clothes, appliances, etc…). Not only that, if you have a trade or skill, you can volunteer your expertise to a person or organization. For me, I. ve supported will and landlord tennat clinic for the needy and given a host legal hours aways every year to family and friends who are in need of legal counsel.

In my opinion, if the people behind the number of social media posts were actually engaged in volunteer activity about what they claim to be so passionate about, the negative effects of the issue they are posting about would probably be at least reduced, if not

eliminated. There are far to many people posting, but not doing anything. If we care about the Syrian refugees, are we donating time or money to the effort to help Syrian refugees? Heroin is harming people at alaerming rate. Are the social media commentators

involved in a cause or group to help reduce the negative impact of heroin? So you. re passionate about green energy, animals, civil rights, or some other social topics? Are you involved in a specific activity to abate the negative impact of what you claim to be so passionate about? We must give back by to the community by engaging in actions to curb the negative side effects of the social and political issues we are most passionate.

Summary

Life success begins with a critical self-assessment. The self-assessment triggers the journey to find our

passion and purpose in life from which our life plans flows
with specific goals underneath

85

that life plan. Once we make this discovery, we have our mission and we must direct our time and energy towards that mission. As we seek to maximize our own potential, we also will be empowered to assist other in the same journey. As we move towards life success with a life plan [next chapter], there is a compelling reason to give back to others. This total view of life success enables us to change society, but not in a boil the ocean mentality, but with measurable impactful behavior with tangible results.

CHAPTER 6:   A LIFE PLAN: SUCCEEDING AT GOALS

" Do or do not, there is no try!" – Yoda

Before we go on any trip, we decide our destination, specific travel itinerary, and means of getting to our destination. And then we pack our bags and go. In planning goals, we should make our goals objectively measurable and few in number. At least every year we should develop and refine our own goals/resolutions. In Wright On My People speak; we refer to as a " Life Plan" . My sons and I have workeda " Life Plan" many years to hold ourselves accountable to our goals. At the end of each year, we evaluate how well we actually performed against the Life Plan and grade ourselves. Here are key excerpts of my 2013 Life Plan:

<u>Ross Wright Life Plan 2013:</u>

o *<u>Short term plan: 2 years or less</u>*
  -big top arch window in living room replaced 2013
  -solar energy ramp up: experimentation small
  devices, batteries to begin process for large
  solar panel install

-begin to set aside down payment funds to acquire
duplex/triplex complex, and put more in 401k (begin
May 2014)[in progress, August 2015]
Malachi and Bilal part time jobs school year 2013,
begin college and work fall 2014 [complete]
Malachi and Bilal high-school grad present trip to
London and Paris June 2014, funded from XU/UC pay
along with other side work.
[complete]

o *Middle term plans 2-5 years*
  -Malachi and Bilal complete or finishing up
  trade school/vocational or college training[on
  target, in progress]
  -obtain BJJ black belt, very close to going to
  brown now[complete late 2014]

o *Long term plans 5+ years*
  -Investigate retirement in a lower cost country near
  US, retain US citizenship and assets in US, rent
  overseas, explore Countries,

-post corporate life, teach at university and run
  consulting business to consult. Business
  transactions worldwide[on target if I elect to do
  so]
  -create charitable trust in name of Patricia D
  Wright and Samuel Ross Wright to promote education,
  and not the traditional, played out theories, but
  new thinking with BJJ and spirituality woven in.
  [complete via trust documents and will]

*In late December 2013, I earned a B on my performance. I then
used the mid-term and long term life plan as my short term plans
for 2014.

My Life Plan helps me stay on track and allocate my time
properly per our discussion on wise use of time in the
previous chapters. And this is the beauty of a Life Plan,
while it keeps us on track; it allows the flexibility to make
mid-stream adjustments. This manner of living is much
smoother to me than whimsically making up new goals every
year, week or day without any true focus or accountability.
We. ve all come across, or maybe we are ˢ that personₑ who
articulates goals, creative ideas and recommendations, but
puts very little energy behind making that goal, creative
idea or
recommendation into a reality.

As we enter that time of the year when we create next
year's goals and resolutions towards our Life Plan, we must
first ask ourselves, "How did we perform against our 2015
goals/resolution?ₑ =Accountability. In order to set a
legitimate goal/resolution, it must be objectively
measurable (not "I'm going to save the world"=not
measurable).

Simply stated in 2015, if your goal was to save $5,000, and you saved $4,500, you did well. If your goal was to lower your cholesterol, blood pressure or weight, that is also measurable by medical instruments/tests and a scale. If your goal was to get a promotion or buy a car, this goals is also measurable. Did it happen?

We can't have open ended goals/resolutions that cannot be measured objectively or else you have a MEANINGLESS goal or resolution. In my case, for the year 2015, here were my key goals [all had specific objective metrics around them]: incorporation of WOMP LLC, raising chickens for eggs, more solar purchases to be less dependent on the grid, providing wisdom advancement of my sons' lives on the road to manhood (education, employment, behaving in a upright manner), marriage if they desire-communication with connectedness to valuded people to set our goals along with integration of health care, retirement planning, new families, new house acquisition, etc...), BJJ World Championships in Vegas, personal savings, financial and investment goals with specific dollar figures and savings amounts, nutrition goals (weight, health numbers).

Measuring my 2015 performance against resolution/goal (married people should measure themselves individually and as a couple), I've rated myself overall a "B" (didn't win Worlds BJJ championships, but competed honorably), could have done better on returns with some investment accounts, acquisition of the two right pieces of real estate ongoing process—money available, but looking for right parcels).

So as we all articulate 2016 goals/resolutions to be rolled into our Life Plan, remember to grade/rate yourself on your 2015 goals/resolutions, discover areas where you did good or bad to improve and then create objectively measurably 2016 goals and resolutions and do the same thing next year. The WOMP resolutions/goals setting process above will ensure focus,
accountability, pats on the back when EARNED, and kicks in the butt when we need to improve and do better.

As the Scriptures teach, the Word is not enough. The Word ³ must become flesh₈ and dwell among us. So the next time you come up with some nifty idea or suggestion, why not take the additional steps to bring that idea into reality from which the world may benefit. Remember, we have the time to do so.

91

I. m sure when Steve Jobs talked about creating an iPad
or the first cell phones were developed or the streaming of
music and/or TV over the internet was discussed, there were
many who may have had the idea before the ultimate inventor
did. However, Bill Gates, Steve Jobs, Mark Zuckerberg and
others had the vision and courage to bring their idea into
reality. We must similarly have that viewpoint on our own
potential. We all have gifts that we can discover and
translate the power of our gifts into this world. It doesn. t
have to always be ᵗ other personᵣ or the magic genie or
person from the sky who is going to fix it all.

Do we ever notice that as we get older, the things in
our life that used to take on great significance become very
insignificant? Why is that? Well, we get the opportunity to
experience life, deaths of family members and friends,
personal health challenges, professional set-backs and other
life challenges that put what we thought was important into
greater perspective. This greater perspective gives us
sharpened clarity and self-awareness that escaped us maybe
just a few years ago. This principle works in concert with
the time accountability concept we. ve discussed and allows
us to hone in on what really matters. Ask yourself this

question occasionally, " What really matters?" And then
assess whether or not your activities and the doing of
those activities reflects what really matters. In many
cases, we will find a gap between our actions and what
really matters, which requires some life re-alignment and
correction.

There was movie I watched some years ago entitled, " The
Adjustment Bureau". The basic plot of the movie is the main
character attempts to win a seat in the U.S. Senate. Just as
he gets in the thick of the political race he realizes he's
romantically falling for a ballerina. As this happens, a
group of mysterious men conspire to keep the two apart. The
main character realizes he is up against the agents of Fate
itself--the men of The Adjustment Bureau--who will do
everything in their considerable power to prevent the
ballerina and main character from being together
romantically. In the face of overwhelming odds, he must
either let her go and accept a predetermined path or risk
everything to defy Fate and be with her.

Not every decision we make in life is that deep or
involves shifting Fate, but there are some critical
navigational turns we make that will have ramifications on

our lives for many, many years. We have to be our own

Adjustment Bureau in reacting to those situations

that may get us off course from our Life Plan developed continuously through introspection and discipline. We must engage in self-
correction with the support of those around us.

The energy we surround ourselves with has an appreciable impact on our mindset and well-being. In movies like Star Wars, there is a phenomenon known as " the Force," which is a neutral repository of energy, which can be used for good (Jedi-Light Side) or evil (Sith-Dark Side). As we construct our Life Plan and embark upon the fulfillment of that plan, we must build the positive Force around us by keeping in our inner circles those who will constructively critique, support, love and push us to our limits to make our Life Plan a reality.

Summary

A life plan is an absolute perquisite to understanding how we can best allocate our precious time in the limited period of time we have on Earth. It is truly sad to see in the eyes of another human being a loss of hope without any real life purpose. This person haphazardly buzzes along from one activity or thing to the next with no true overall focus to direct their lives. As a promoter of individual freedom, I respect people who may want to live this way, but in my opinion, you can see their yearning to accomplish something bigger. However, the life drifter has no focus and is unable to find their way.

Instead of annual New Year resolutions, which are fleeting and often ignored as the year progresses, the Life Plan imposes upon us a continuous evaluative mechanism to check our progress along the way and to adapt or modify our life plan as thing unfolds. I believe 14 years old is about the right age to draft our first Life Plan. There are 8,760 hours in a year. Surely, we can dedicate two hours per month (January-November), and four hours during December to developing, evaluating and revising our life plan (26 hours out of 8,760 per year). Life is a fantastic journey. We must make the most of the time we are given, have fun, live with zest and leave a great legacy for the next generation. Wright On My People!

Bibliography

1. Facebook, IMF 2014 "Facebook users Compared to China and India Populations"
2. Holy Bible
3. Holy Quran
4. Pew Research Center June-Sept, 2014 "Changing Religious Landscape" 5. Pew Research Center, "The World. s religious make-up"
6. Pew Research Center, "Life Satisfaction: % of people rating their life satisfaction between 7-10", 2014
7. "How it ends: From You to the Universe", W.W. Norton & Company, April 2011
8. Harvard Business Review ("Executives, Protect Your Alone Time", December 16, 2015)
9. "Happiness and GDP", Ipsos; International Monetary Fund (IMF)
10. "Cautious Borrowing", New York Federal Reserve Bank via Wall Street Journal 2015
11. "Loneliness May Warp Our Genes, And Our Immune Systems", National Public Radio November 29, 2015)
12. "How to spot malnutrition and how to remedy it", Wall Street Journal via Alliance to Advance Patient Nutrition
13. "Dueling Diets; Heavy Burden", Wall Street Journal via Dr. Kelly Ann Petrucci US Department of Agriculture
14. "Something for Nothing: Participation in Volunteer Time", Charities Aid Foundation 2012
15. "Homegrown Extremism", New American Foundation 2015
16. Denzel Washington to College Grads: "Put God First in Everything You Do. . Relevant Magazine, May 11, 2015. Read more at http://www.relevantmagazine.com/slices/denzel-washington-college-grads-put-god-first-everything-you-do#mOYoOtjhgVlY3rEw.99

<u>[In no order of preference and not only these books]</u>:

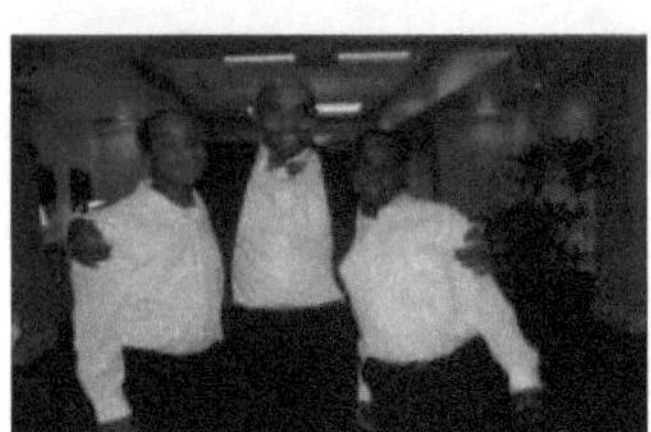

1. ꝅ The Art of Hanging Loose in a Uptight Worldꝅ by Dr. Ken Olson

2.   ꝅ Atlas Shruggedꝅ by Ayn

3.   Rand

4.   ꝅ Beowulfꝅ by Anonymous

5.   Poet

Krishnamurti

6. ꝅ Multipliers: How the Best Leaders Make Everyone Smarterꝅ by Liz Wiseman & Greg McKweon

7.   ꝅ The Alchemistꝅ by
                             Paulo Coehlo

8.   ꝅ The Seven Spiritual
                             Laws of Successꝅ by

9.   Deepok Chopra ꝅ The
                             Millionaire Next Doorꝅ

10.   by Thomas J. Stanley

Thank you for your kind support of our book!

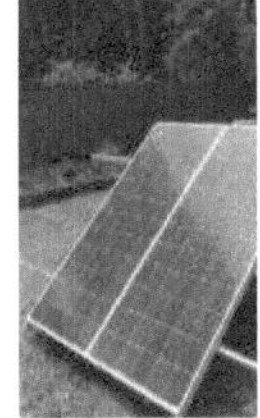
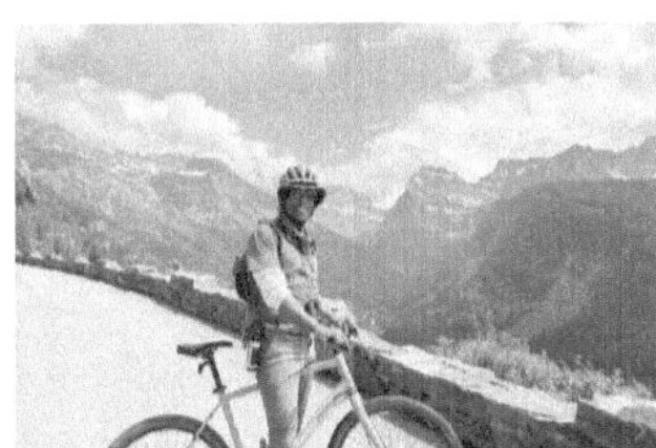
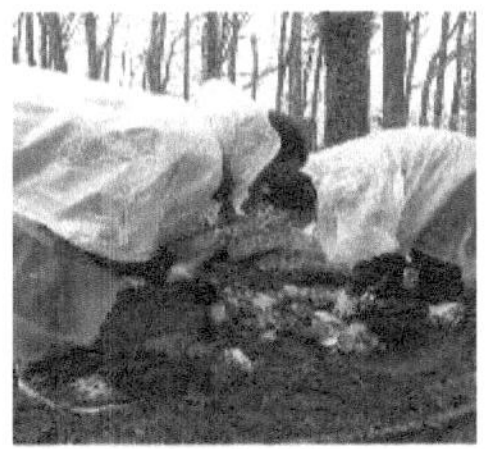
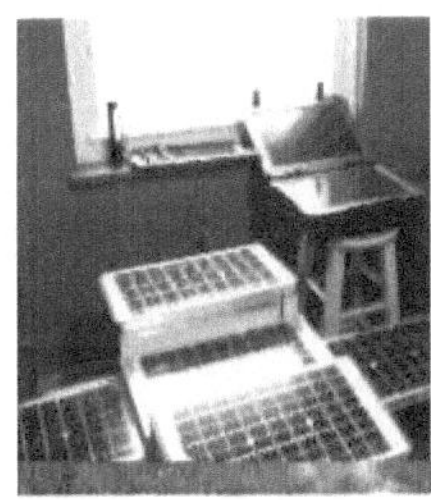
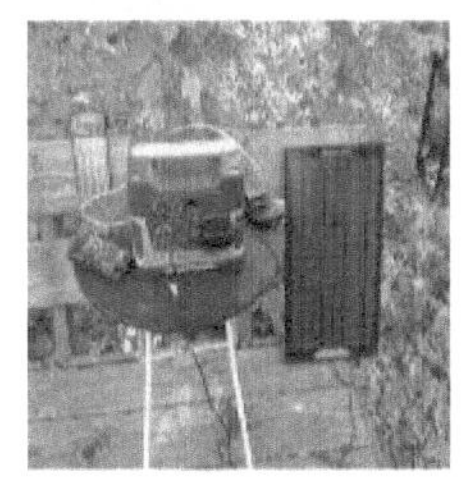
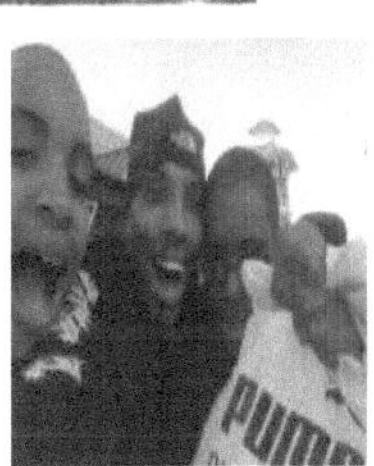
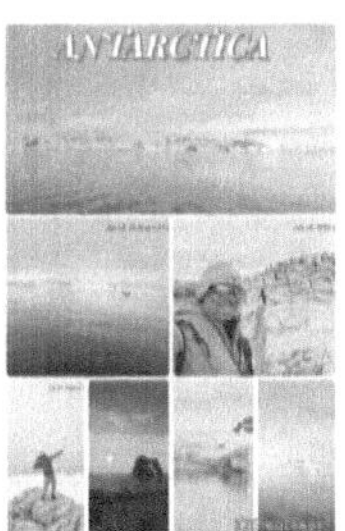